EARTH-CLOSETS

AND

EARTH SEWAGE.

BY

GEORGE E. WARING, JR.

(of Ogden Farm),

AUTHOR OF "EARTH-CLOSETS, HOW TO MAKE THEM AND HOW TO USE THEM," "DRAINING FOR PROFIT, AND DRAINING FOR HEALTH," "THE ELEMENTS OF AGRICULTURE," AND "THE HANDY-BOOK OF HUSBANDRY;" FORMERLY AGRICULTURAL ENGINEER OF THE CENTRAL PARK, NEW YORK.

ILLUSTRATED.

PRICE FIFTY CENTS.

NEW YORK:

THE TRIBUNE ASSOCIATION,

154 NASSAU STREET.

1870.

EARTH-CLOSET COMPANY.

LOCAL OFFICES.

Boston	19 Doane Street	J. Gardiner White.
New York	597 Broadway	H. P. Gray, Jr.
Philadelphia	513 Market Street	E. R. Bowen.
Baltimore	1 Holliday Street	W. A. Bryant & Co.
Washington	910 Pennsylvania Avenue	E. Eveleth.
New Orleans	2 Carondelet Street	Dr. J. J. Castellanos.
Memphis	273 Main Street	H. T. Aborn.
Chicago	138 La Salle Street	James Waring.
Ohio, Western Pennsylvania, etc.	Massillon, Ohio	John Hoskin.
Albany	82 State Street	C. H. Strong.

AGENCIES.

Bangor, Maine—Dole Brothers.
Newport, R. I.—Swinburne, Peckham & Co.
West Winsted, Conn.—David W. Coe.
New Haven, Conn.—Dry Earth Co., 289 Chapel Street.
Bridgeport, Conn.—T. B. Doolittle.
So. Norwalk, Conn.—F. H. Nash & Bro.
Stamford, Conn.—J. L. Lockwood.
Plainfield, N. J.—John T. Lee.
Tenafly, N. J.—Thos. C. Veal.
Burlington, N. J.—R. B. Carter.
Pottsville, Penn.—Bright & Co.
Bradford, Penn.—F. A. Newell.
Pittsburg, Penn.—E. J. Seibert.
Greenville, Penn.—Packard & Co.
Alexandria, Va.—Green & Bro.
Lexington, Va.—Fuller & Sloan.
Norfolk, Va.—Thos. R. Gary & Co.
Wheeling, W. Va.—Metcalf & Burt.
Portsmouth, Ohio—John McGinley.
Indianapolis, Indiana—Amos F. Fay.
Louisville, Ky.—Speed, Magens & Co.
Nashville, Tenn.—Maney & Shaifer.
Morris, Illinois.—E. Sanford.
Milwaukee, Wis.—Geo. B. Kellogg & Co., 115 Wisconsin Street.
Minneapolis, Minn.—Charles Darrow.
Hot Springs, Ark.—Dr. O. B. Knode.
Providence, R. I.—W. C. Townsend, 70 Weybosset Street.
Burlington, Vt.—E. E. Ryer.
Lyndonville, Vt.—N. P. Lovering, Jr.
Pittsfield, Mass.—M. O. Hutchings & Co.
River Head, N. Y.—Charles Hallett.
Yonkers, N. Y.—C. F. Hanby.
Fishkill Landing, N. Y.—W. H. Van Wagenen.
Poughkeepsie, N. Y.—A. Cannon, Jr.
Rhinebeck, N. Y.—Wm. Carroll.
Troy, N. Y.—Carter & Ford.
Schenectady, N. Y.—Jacob De Forest.
Cambridge, N. Y.—Dr. T. C. Wallace.
Potsdam, N. Y.—Batchelder & Son.
Binghamton, N. Y.—L. L. Olmsted.
Elmira, N. Y.—Robinson's Furniture Rooms.
Rochester, N. Y.—Porter & Chapin.
Staten Island, North Side, all of the landings.
Vanderbilt Landing, Staten Island—James R. Robinson.
Watertown, N. Y.—J. Felt.
Faribault, Minn.—S. H. Jaques.
Columbia, S. C.—Alex. Y. Lee.
Magnolia, E. Florida.—Dr. S. Rogers.
York, Penn.—A. B. Farquhar.
Battle Creek, Mich.—John Butcher
Richmond, Va.—C. W. Harrison.
Hillsdale, Mich.—J. W. Winsor & Sons.
Dubuque, Iowa—John Hunter.
Omaha, Neb.—E. K. Abbott, 506 13th St.

EARTH-CLOSETS

AND

EARTH SEWAGE.

BY

GEORGE E. WARING, JR. (of Ogden Farm).

INCLUDING:

THE EARTH SYSTEM (DETAILS).
THE MANURE QUESTION.
SEWAGE AND CESS-POOL DISEASES.
THE DRY-EARTH SYSTEM FOR CITIES AND TOWNS.
THE DETAILS OF EARTH SEWAGE.
THE PHILOSOPHY OF THE EARTH SYSTEM.

SEVENTEEN ILLUSTRATIONS.

NEW YORK:
THE TRIBUNE ASSOCIATION,
154 NASSAU STREET.

1870.

CONTENTS.

THE EARTH SYSTEM.

IT is barely two years since the first complete description of the Earth-Closet was published in America—in Judd's Agricultural Annual for 1868—and not a year and a half since the first Commode was imported; yet it may already be said that the Earth-Closet has gained such a foot-hold that its universal adoption (except in houses in which there are water-closets supplied from public water-works) is certain. It has now reached the "important if true" stage. The whole community is ready to concede that, if the Dry Earth system will accomplish what is claimed for it, nothing can prevent its general adoption. It remains necessary only to prove that it will do this, which, with the facts at command, is an easy task.

When my previous pamphlet* was written, I could adduce no evidence except that published by the English company in its advertising circular, and the single trial in my own house. I am now, fortunately, supplied with the most conclusive testimony from various parts of this country, some of which is even stronger than anything from England or India. My own opportunities for observation and experience have been excellent, and I am more than ever convinced that no better service can be rendered to the country than in extending among all classes of its people a knowledge of the inestimable advantages of the new system. I speak thus strongly, because I am sure all thought-

* Earth Closets: How to Make Them and How to Use Them.

ful persons will admit that the facts herein set forth are ample justification for any enthusiasm on the subject.

Precisely what the Earth-Closet and its accessories, as now contrived, accomplish is the following:

1. A comfortable closet on any floor of the house, supplied with earth, and cleansed of its deposits without the intervention or knowledge of any member of the household.

2. A portable commode in any dressing-room, bedroom, or closet, the care of which is no more disagreeable than is that of an anthracite stove.

3. Appliances for the use of immovable invalids which entirely remove the distressing accompaniments of their care.

4. The complete and effectual removal of all the liquid wastes of sleeping-rooms and kitchen.

5. The utilizing of a manure worth (including kitchen and laundry wastes) at least $10 per annum for each member of the family, old and young.

6. The removal of the most fertile source of typhoid fever and dysentery, and the prevention of cholera infection.

7. The complete suppression of the odors which, despite the comfort and elegance of modern living, still hang about our cess-pools and privy-vaults, and attend the removal of their contents.

I have excepted houses which are supplied with water by public works from those into which the Earth-Closet may be expected to find its way immediately; but I am confident that the second, third, fifth, and sixth of the above specified advantages will, in due time, give the Dry Earth Commode at least an accessory place even in such houses; and I believe that these advantages, together with the question of cost, will revolutionize the sewage question, and that public sewers will, in future, be restricted to the removal of liquid drainage only.

The cost of the introduction of the Earth-Closet system is trifling when compared with its benefits. For instance: A two-story country house can be supplied with a closet on each floor for the use of the members of the family, one near the kitchen for the use of servants, a movable commode for use in the sick-room, and conveniences for the disposal of the entire liquid wastes of the house, all so arranged as to require but a trifling amount of attention—less even than with the water-closet system—for about $250.

A commode alone, which is ample, with a daily renewal of the earth, for the use of eight persons, costs about $30, and for the same amount a stationary closet may be put up in any unoccupied room, which will hold enough earth to last this number of persons a month or six weeks.

Nor need the benefits that the earth system offers be confined even to those who can afford this moderate cost, for this is necessary only for the sake of convenience. Any process by which the evacuations are immediately enveloped in dry earth or dry coal-ashes will accomplish the purpose, and the poorest cabin in the land may, absolutely without cost, be supplied with some provision that will obviate the necessity for its invalids and its women to expose themselves in inclement weather.

The following paper on the Earth-Closet, written for the New Haven *Palladium*, by Prof. S. W. Johnson, of Yale College, is entitled to the most careful attention, not only on account of the reputation of its author, but because of the practical way in which it sets forth the leading advantages of the earth system:

"There are two grave questions which enforce attention from "every dweller in the city, and should not be neglected by those who "have the country for their home. These questions relate to the dispo-"sition of the liquid and solid waste of the human body. One of them "is, How shall the waste be effectually prevented from being an annoy-"ance and source of disease? and the other, How shall it be made a "means of fertility to the soil, and thus an item of national wealth?

"The annoyance that results from want of care in putting our *exuviæ* "out of the way is not often encountered among us in the public manner "that is common in the old countries, where poverty and necessity have "made people less fastidious than we are. We do not establish our "privies in our front halls or next the staircases of our houses, and the "openings of our sewers do not send forth the choking stench that "nearly prostrates the stranger walking by, as is the case in many a Ger-"man city. We provide well-ventilated temples in our groves and gar-"dens in honor of Stercutius, or by the costly aid of plumber and potter "furnish water transportation by a speedy route to some dark grotto of "earth or ocean cave, and this is well as far as it goes. But our poor "are already in their own filth, and, as our towns enlarge and build more "densely, the well-to-do, and even the rich, must, sooner or later, be "swamped in the impurities of their own and of past generations.

"Nothing is better established than the connection between human "excrement and certain fearful epidemics.

"It is on all hands admitted that cholera is most frequently and "certainly transmitted to healthy persons by the intestinal evacuations of "those who have been sick with this disease. The instance of the out-"break of this malady in a country town of Maine, that followed the un-"packing of a sailor's chest containing the soiled garments that eight "months before had served in his last hours on the other side of the "globe, is but one of a multitude that settle this point.

"Typhoid fever, a form of disease very prevalent among us, is "often traceable, with scarcely less certainty, to privy-vaults, cess-pools, "and sewers. It is stated that Prince Albert, of England, probably con-"tracted the disease that was fatal to him, from the foul air that found "its way into his study out of a forgotten sewer through a crack in the "wall.

"Most often it is our drinking-water that brings into us the conta-"mination. New Haven is built upon a gravel plain, and the open soil "gives free passage to the liquids that fall upon it. In multitudes of "cases, the well is but a few yards or feet from a cess-pool that receives "the kitchen slops on one hand, and a privy-vault on the other. Earth "has a remarkable power of absorption and disinfection, but this power "chiefly resides in its fine and impalpable portions—in the clay and not "in the coarse particles of sand. A well, distant fifty feet horizontally "from a privy-vault, both in a clayey soil, the writer knows which has "yielded excellent drinking-water for thirty years, as attested by its taste, "and by the fact that for that period no case of fever occurred on the "premises. The writer knows another well, similarly situated in New "Haven, which furnished good water for about five years after it was ex-"cavated, in what was until then a vacant lot, but after this interval be-

"came unpleasant in taste, its flavor plainly suggesting the nature of its "impurities.

"In his researches on the cholera, in Bavaria, in 1854, Pettenkofer "traced its spread in several cases, in the most indubitable manner, to "the use of water which had been in contact with the fæces of "cholera patients.

"The use of open vaults or water-closets emptying in cess-pools "tends to fill up the soil with fæcal matter. A single vault poisons a "circumscribed space around it. External to this limit the filth is "destroyed by the action of the oxygen of the air, which is the great pu- "rifier. Within the limit named, the animal matters preponderate either "constantly or at some period of the year. They may long remain sim- "ply disagreeable without being dangerous, and may again, of a sudden, "in a way whose details have as yet escaped investigation, become "the seed-bed or the nursery of the infection that breaks out in fevers "and dysentery. The danger increases as the quantity of filth and the "number of its receptacles increase. To cover them up does not neces- "sarily remove the evil. The putrid matters soak into the soil, and move "upward and downward in it with the motion of the soil-water. When "we have copious rains, they are carried down perhaps to nearly the "level of the water in our wells. In the heat and drought of August, "these matters rise again. In the absence of rain, the rapid drying "of the surface creates an upward capillary flow of the ground-water. "The matters which in rainy times follow the surface-water to the "depths, in drought follow the ground-water to the surface.

"The safest mode of escaping the evils in question hitherto adopted "in closely built towns consists in removing all human excreta to a dis- "tance by subterranean sewerage. In paved cities, the street hydrants, "which with the rains wash the surface filth into a system of under- "drains, and the water-closets which connect every house with the same, "would seem to offer every immunity against the accumulation of fæcal "matters. The immunity is, in fact, very considerable in those cases "where the system is well carried out; where the water supply is suffi- "ciently copious, and the sewage is promptly carried off to the sea. "There always remain the objections that poverty cannot and indo- "lence will not 'make the connections,' that sewers will leak, and "rivers and harbors are made noisome with the rottenness that is poured "into them.

"The waste involved in the 'civilized' way of treating the materials "under notice is immense. Every harvest brings from the country to the "city, from the West to the East, vast bulk of beef, corn, and hay, whose "use to the city people does not for the most part consist in any perma- "nent giving of its elements, but which, after having weighted the wheel "of life through half a turn and dropped off as waste, admits of conver- "sion into food again, if but carried back to the fields. The gardeners "and farmers in our immediate vicinity are obliged to disburse heavy "sums each year for the phosphates and nitrogen which their crops de- "mand, and which their land cannot adequately supply. The guanoes "and fish-manures which are brought from a distance or manufactured "at heavy cost for their use are in reality paid for not by them, but by "those who purchase their produce in the city markets. The animal "who stands at the head of creation requires the richest food, and yields "to the food-producer the richest return. It requires but little art to "convert his excrement into increment, and the conversion may be "made extremely profitable.

"In countries where the thing has been tried, it has been found "that the annual evacuations of a well-fed man suffice to manure half an "acre of ground, and their fertilizing value may be safely stated at $5. "Indeed, if put into a suitable form as regards dryness and texture, they "would compete with our standard fertilizers at twice this sum. We are "told, in fact, that formerly they were valued at $9, gold, in Flan- "ders, and it is hardly to be supposed that they have fallen in esti- "mation.

"The writer has it from undoubted authority that the Chinese agri- "culturists near Fuh-Chau will give a day's work for ten gallons of urine; "and it is well understood that the teeming population of China and "Japan could not subsist if they wasted this means of enriching the soil, "as do we and most other of the 'barbarians' west of the Celestial and "Flowery Kingdoms.

"If it be true that the value of the waste in question amounts to "but one-third of the sum above named per head annually for the entire "population, old and young, then not less than $80,000 is every year "lost to New Haven; for of all this treasure next to nothing is ever "saved, on account of its excessive proneness to decomposition. To "economize this fertilizer, it must either be used after no long interval, as "is the Chinese practice, or it must be dried and disinfected when per- "fectly fresh. All attempts to accomplish this result by manufacturing "or chemical processes, involving carriage of the fresh material, have "signally failed.

"The means of satisfying at once all demands of sanitary science "and of agriculture is, however, fortunately everywhere at hand, and of "extreme simplicity and cheapness in its application. *Dry and fine earth* "is the material.

"This property of earth is no new discovery. Its use was pre-"scribed to the Israelites (Deuteronomy xxiii. 12 and 13), and is turned "to good account by the instincts of our domestic carnivora. The Rev. "Henry Moule, an English clergyman, was the first to elaborate, by a "careful study of the subject, a plan for the systematic employment of "earth for this purpose. In 1858, he published a pamphlet entitled "'National Health and Wealth,' and in 1863 he contributed, to the "'Journal of the Royal Agricultural Society of England,' a paper headed "'Earth *versus* Water for the Removal and Utilization of Excrementi-"tious Matter.' In these publications, he pointed out the fact that, "First, a very small portion of dry and sifted earth (1½ pints) is suffi-"cient, by covering the deposit, to arrest effluvium, to prevent fermen-"tation (which so soon sets in when water is used), and the conse-"quent generation and emission of noxious gases. Secondly, that, if "within a few hours, or even a few days, the mass which would "be formed by the repeated layers of deposit be intimately mixed "by a coarse rake or spade, or by a mixer made for the purpose, "then in five or ten minutes neither to the eye nor sense of "smell is anything perceptible but so much earth. He found, "further, that, 'when about three cart-loads of sifted earth had "been used for a family which averaged fifteen persons, and left "under a shed, the material first employed was sufficiently dried to be "used again. This process of alternate mixing and drying was re-"newed five times, the earth still retaining its absorbent powers appar-"ently unimpaired. Of the visitors taken to the spot, none could guess "the nature of the compost, though in some cases the heap which they "visited in the afternoon had been turned over the same morning.'

"'Three cart-loads of earth served fifteen persons for half a year, "being used five times over in that time.' 'At Bradford-on-Avon, the "same earth having been dried and used repeatedly at the school of "the union-house, in which there are fifty-five children, the whole com-"post did not exceed a cart-load and a half, or thirty cwt., at the end of "five months.'

"The arrangements required to constitute an earth-closet are not "necessarily complex or expensive. It is only needful that a space be "had below the privy-seat, the bottom of which should be of flagging or "cement, and a little above the ground level, or at least protected from

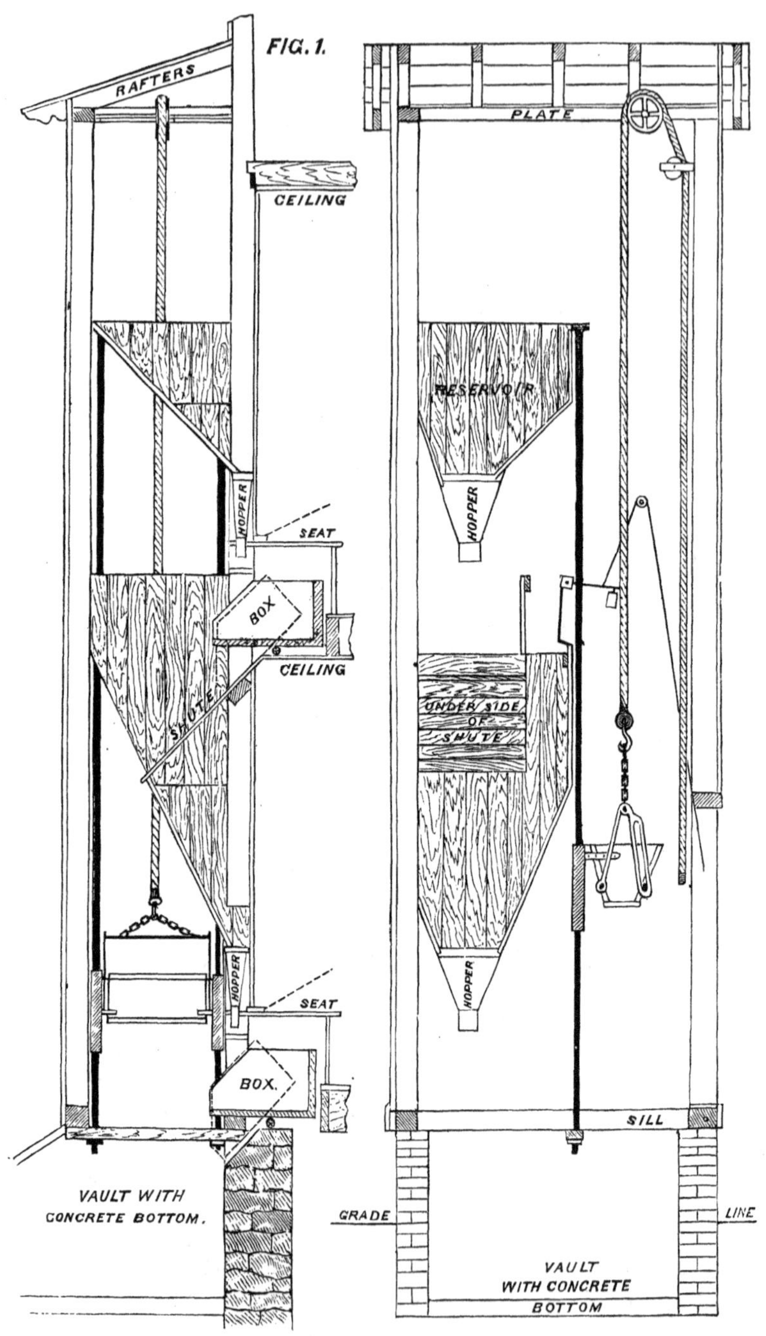

PLAN OF CLOSETS ON TWO FLOORS,

WITH HOIST AND DUMP.

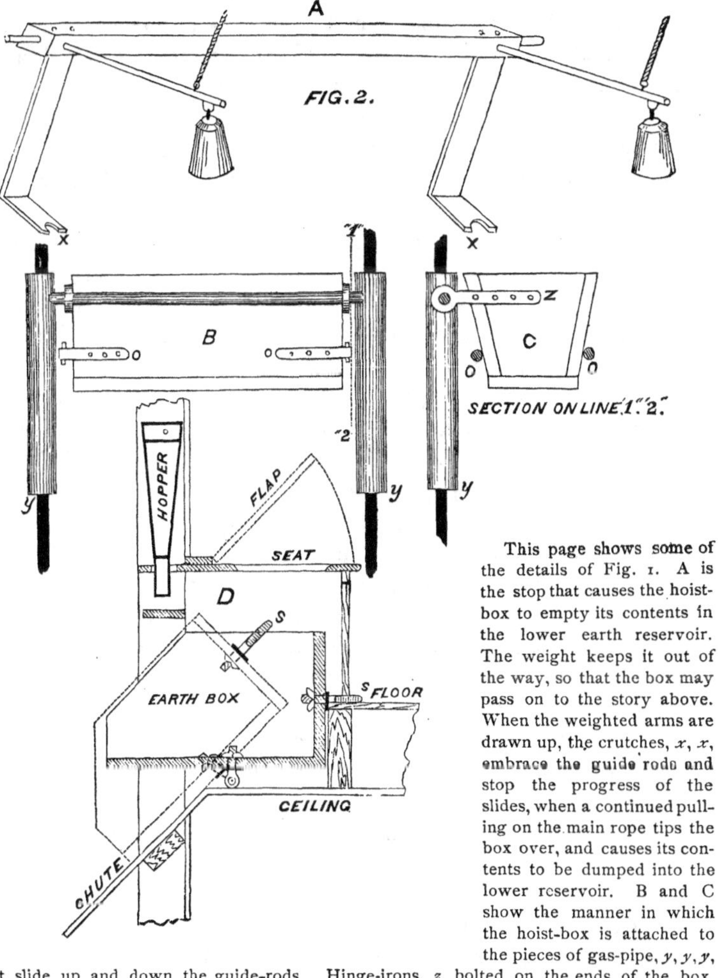

This page shows some of the details of Fig. 1. A is the stop that causes the hoist-box to empty its contents in the lower earth reservoir. The weight keeps it out of the way, so that the box may pass on to the story above. When the weighted arms are drawn up, the crutches, *x*, *x*, embrace the guide rods and stop the progress of the slides, when a continued pulling on the main rope tips the box over, and causes its contents to be dumped into the lower reservoir. B and C show the manner in which the hoist-box is attached to the pieces of gas-pipe, *y*, *y*, *y*, that slide up and down the guide-rods. Hinge-irons, *z*, bolted on the ends of the box, connect it with a rod between the slides (which passes through the eyes of the hinges). The box is suspended (as shown in Fig. 1) by the ears, *o*, *o*. The movement is directly upward, until the slides strike the stop on either story, then the continued strain causes the hinges to revolve around the rod between them, until the box is tipped over and thrown forward over the edge of the reservoir. D shows the construction of the tray under the seat. This tray has no back end, and when it is tilted its contents are thrown down the shute. When the tray is brought back to its place, it is held there by closing the door of the riser, which locks the pin, *s*, into a notch in the sill.

In Fig. 1, the shute from the second story closet occupies a portion of the space that would otherwise be given to the reservoir of the first story. This reservoir, however, is wider than the shute, and is continued up beside it.

The vault may be on the surface of the ground, or in an excavation, as is preferred. It *must* be tight at the sides and bottom.

" the wet of rain and of the ground. This space should communicate " with a shed at the rear of the privy, to hold on one side a load or two " of dry fine earth (not sand) or sifted coal-ashes, and leave an equal " room unoccupied on the other. Daily, or as often as need be, the " droppings are covered with enough of the dry earth to absorb all liquid, " and, when the space is filled, the mass is hauled out, raked over, and " thrown to one side.

" When the whole has been once used, it may be put through a " second time. If the seat be so constructed that everything falls clear " to the bottom, it may be within the dwelling, and even be warmed by " a register, or otherwise, without danger or unpleasantness. It may be " placed on an upper floor, or a seat may be arranged for every floor. " It is, however, then important that each rise from the seat should be " promptly followed by a dash of earth. The patent fixtures of Mr. " Moule, to be had of the Earth-Closet Company, provide for this, it being " simply needful that a supply of earth be laid in, in a suitable reservoir, " which need not, however, be raised above the ground-floor. For hos- " pital or sick-room use, either a simple commode or pail, with a hod of " earth to apply, or the self-acting commodes of Mr. Moule, may be used.

" Very important it is that hotels, schools, and, we may add, col- " leges, should be provided with this labor and health saving arrange- " ment. In large schools, it is sufficient to put the application of earth in " charge of an attendant. In hotels, the self-acting apparatus is better.

" The fertilizing value of the properly managed compost should be " abundant remuneration to parties supplying earth, especially as its car- " riage is not attended with the slightest odor, and requires not the cover " of darkness to mitigate its terrors, while its use is less disagreeable than " that of Peruvian or fish guano, and not worse than the employment of " any old compost.

" Reader, you should lose no time in providing yourself, and inciting " your neighbor to provide, some form of earth-closet in lieu of the vault " which has hitherto sufficed. Health and economy both demand it! " City authorities, you would do well to enact that all privies within a hun- " dred feet of dwellings, or of wells in use, should be converted into earth- " closets, and to provide for their systematic and thorough inspection."

The great point aimed at in all devices for the improvement of private closets is to make them more comfortable and convenient. But few people think of the loss of fertilizing matter, or of the danger of infection. To the masses these points have no significance. The water-closet has won its way to universal favor on the grounds of convenience, comfort, and decency alone. These it secures; and there is no luxury connected with modern living that is so highly prized by those who have once known its benefits. The water-closet is the chief thing of which women living in the country envy their city cousins the possession. In country-houses, one of the first steps toward elegance is the erection of an expensive water-closet in the house, provided with a force-pump that is doomed to break both the back and the temper of the hired man; a tank and pipes which are pretty sure to be burst by frost every winter; the annual tax of the plumber's bill; and, worse than all, a receptacle in the garden known as a "cess-pool," which usually has a private subterranean communication with the well from which drinking-water is taken. The manure is, of course, lost; it is worse than lost. Too far below the surface to be of use to vegetation, it lies, a festering mass, sending its foul and poisonous gases back through the soil-pipe and kitchen-sink drain into the house, and developing in its putrid fermentation the germs of typhoid fever and dysentery that any film of gravel in the lower soil may carry to the well or the spring.

These drawbacks are of no account as affecting the popularity of the water-closet, for the simple reason that they do not present themselves to the apprehension of the public. Unknown evils are unfeared; and even our best people have a comfortable way of ascribing to the inscrutable dispensations of a Divine Providence rather than to their own folly even such a disease as typhoid fever, *of which no single case ever occurred in a civilized community without the direct intervention of human agency.* The disease is always brought about by our own neglect; and we are to look for the hand of Providence not in its propagation, but rather in our miraculous escape from the traps which we ourselves have set.

If, then, we are to look mainly to the inoffensiveness, accessibility, and comfort of the water-closet for its popularity, we shall recognize the fact that the Earth-Closet can never achieve success unless it offers the

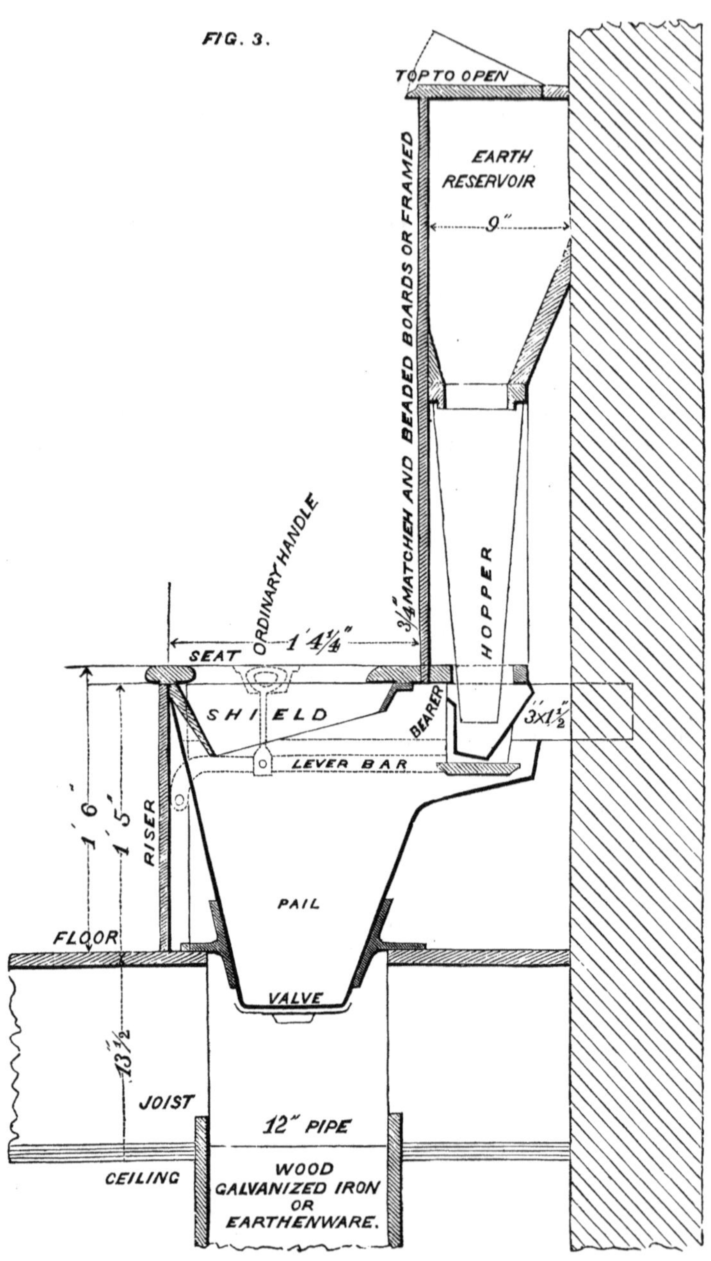

APPARATUS FOR UP-STAIRS CLOSET, WITH VALVED PAIL.

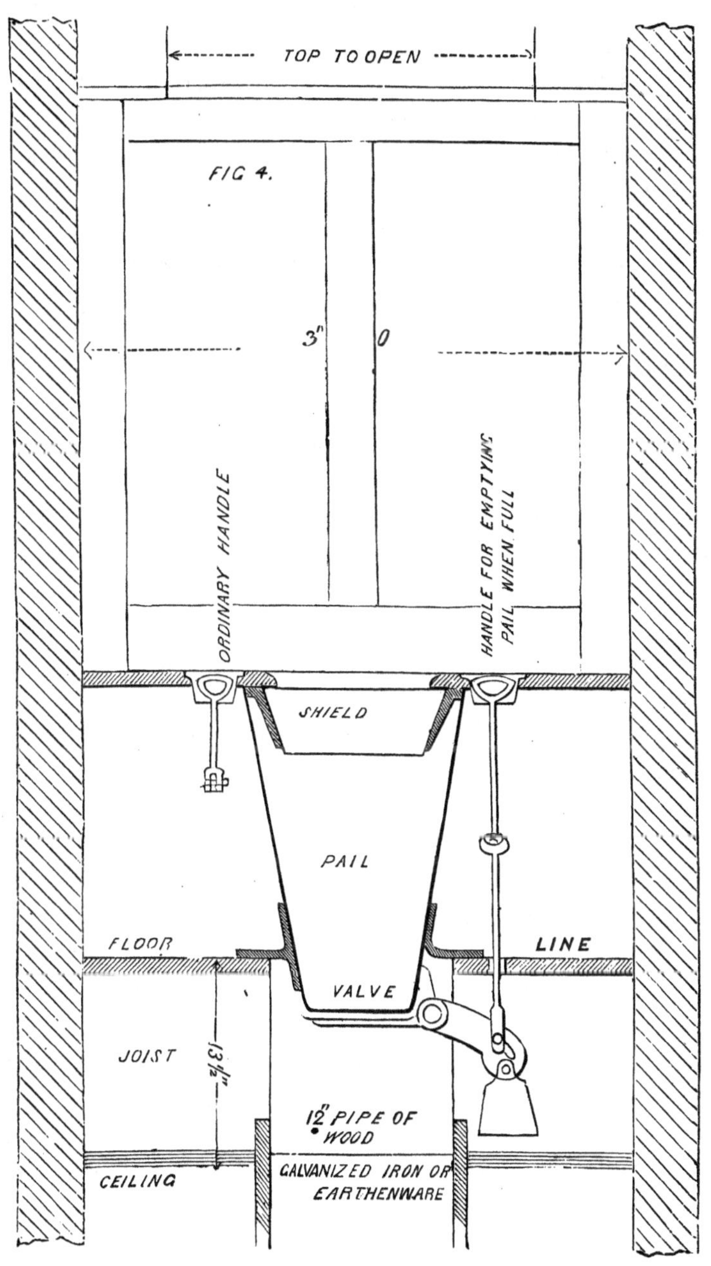

APPARATUS FOR UP-STAIRS CLOSET, WITH VALVED PAIL.

same advantages. It does this, and more. A properly constructed Earth-Closet may be kept in constant use in an occupied room. It is absolutely free from odor. There is an entire absence of the depressing, headachy effect that always accompanies the water-closet or night-chair. A water-closet could not be kept in constant use in a bedroom or sitting-room without injury to the health. An Earth-Closet can be so kept, and herein lies its great superiority simply as a matter of convenience.

This fact being assumed, (and the testimonials contained in this volume establish it,) it becomes a simple question of cost and convenience in what part of the house the Closet shall be placed. Of course, for obvious reasons, its position must be a retired one; but it has the great advantage that it need not be remote, and may be kept within that part of the house that is comfortably warmed. It is, of course, most desirable, as far as the ladies of the family are concerned, that the Closet should be on the second floor of the house, if only one is made. Ordinarily it will be best to build it in one of the outer walls, in order that its earth-shaft may be reached without entering the house. But sometimes this is impossible, and it becomes necessary to carry the soil-pipe directly through the first story, discharging into the cellar. These two plans are shown, the first in Figs. 1 and 2, and the second in Figs. 3, 4, 5, and 6.

For use in farm-houses or other establishments where the services of a man can be commanded occasionally, there is no objection to the arrangement shown in Figs. 3, 4, 5, and 6. The reservoir above the hopper, which may be made to hold a supply of earth for one month or for six months, as may be desired, can be filled in a short time from bags, in which the dry earth may be easily and neatly carried to them. The soil-pipe, which may be built of vitrified pipe, wood, brick, or any other material, discharges into a bin in the cellar, from which the deposit may be readily removed, or where it may lie until dry enough to sift for a second use.*

* I have recently seen, in a cellar in New York, a series of large boxes standing at the side of an Earth-Closet, in which the earth was being dried for repeated use, as a test. One lot had been used six times, and it was impossible, either by its odor or its appearance, to dis-

For towns, however, whether large or small, the convenience of earth supply and removal will probably make it necessary to adopt the plan shown in Figs. 1 and 2. In thickly settled communities, it will be necessary to have some regular system of earth supply and removal that will relieve individual householders not only of the labor and personal attention necessary, but even of all thought concerning it. There are various ways in which this can be done. None has been suggested to me which seems more easily practicable than that proposed by Messrs. Olmsted, Vaux & Co. for the village of Riverside, near Chicago, which is thus described in the *Evening Post:*

"Until the subject was taken in hand by Mr. Olmsted, it was at-
"tended with certain drawbacks, such as the necessity for the house-
"holder to give his personal attention to the supplying of dry earth and
"the removing of deposits, and the possible difficulties with servants on
"the subject of attending to closets on the upper floors of the house.
"By Mr. Olmsted's plan, the closets for the different stories are placed
"directly over each other, and they communicate with a vertical shaft, a
"few feet square, outside of the house. This is the channel by which
"the dry earth is hoisted up, and down which the deposits are dis-
"charged by tilting the trays under the seats on the different stories, an
"operation which may be performed in a moment by any one. The
"vertical shaft has a shallow vault at the bottom for receiving deposits,
"and is provided with a hoisting apparatus with a self-dumping arrange-
"ment, by which the earth-reservoirs on the different floors may be sup-
"plied by a person operating from below. Of the details of the arrange-
"ment for preventing the closets on the different floors from interfering
"with each other, it is only necessary to say that they seem simple and
"complete. There is no door opening from any part of the house into
"the vertical shaft; the only access to it is by a door opening into a back
"yard. This door is to be kept locked, and its key will be in the pocket
"of the public dustman, whose duty it is at stated intervals to make his
"rounds, with his load of sacks filled with dry earth, and his implements
"for removing the contents of the vault. He first fills the different reser-
"voirs, putting in much or little as may be required, but filling them full;

tinguish it from that which had not been used at all. The experimenter expressed his belief that he should be able to use it twelve times, after which he could sell it for over $20 per barrel. In this room, where the closet was in use, and different samples of earth were in various stages of preparation, there was absolutely no offensive odor.

FIG. 5.

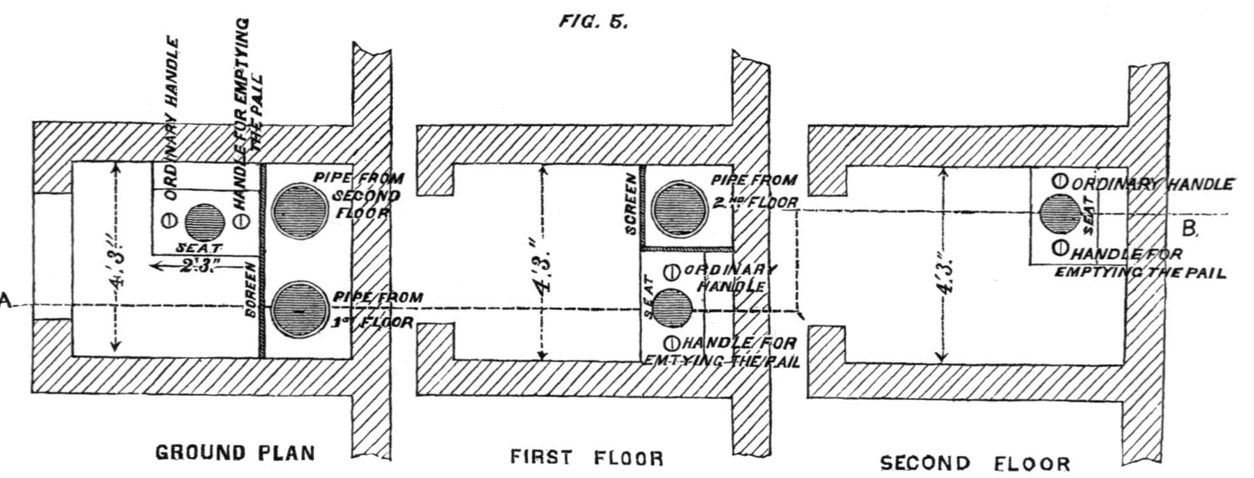

PLAN OF CLOSETS ON THREE FLOORS.

ELEVATION AND SECTION SHOWN IN FIG. 6.

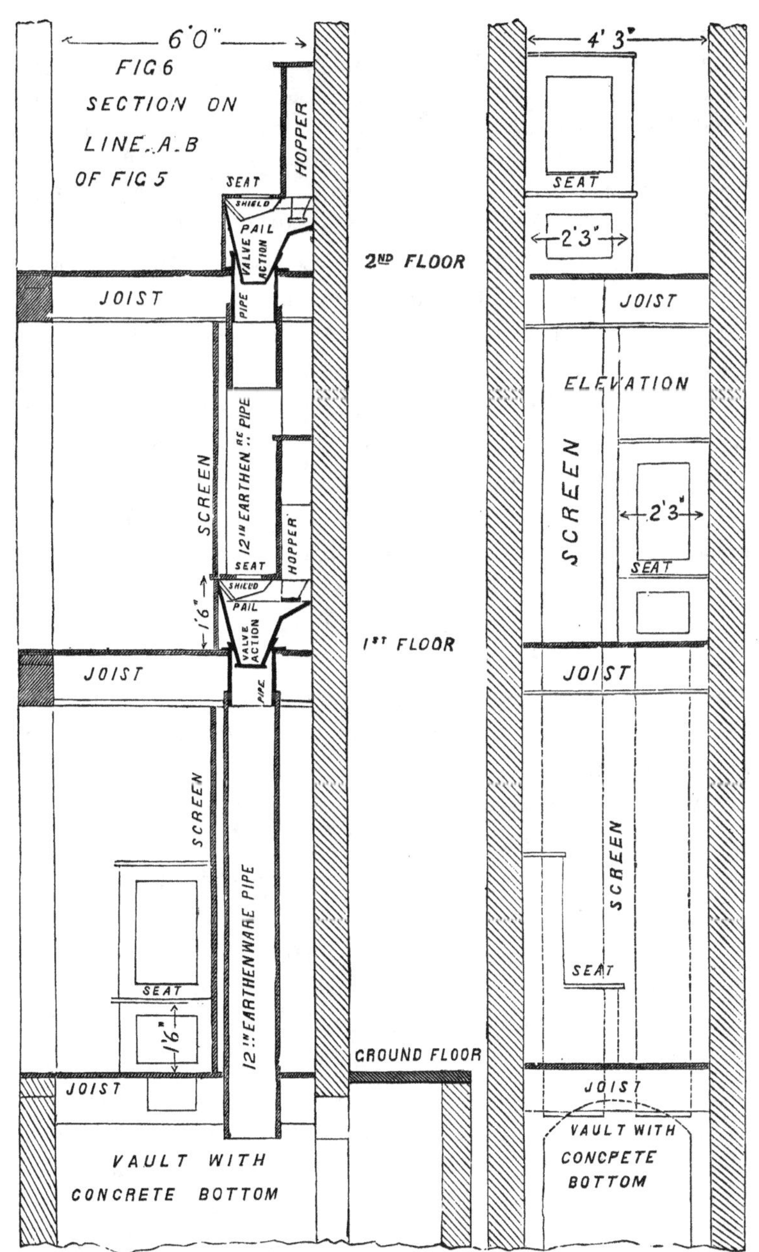
6'0"
FIG 6
SECTION ON
LINE A.B
OF FIG 5
HOPPER
SEAT
SHIELD
PAIL
VALVE ACTION
2ND FLOOR
JOIST
PIPE
12IN EARTHENWARE PIPE
SCREEN
HOPPER
SEAT
SHIELD
1'6"
PAIL
VALVE ACTION
1ST FLOOR
JOIST
PIPE
SCREEN
12IN EARTHENWARE PIPE
SEAT
1'6"
GROUND FLOOR
JOIST
VAULT WITH
CONCRETE BOTTOM
4' 3"
SEAT
2'3"
JOIST
ELEVATION
SCREEN
2'3"
SEAT
JOIST
SCREEN
SEAT
JOIST
VAULT WITH
CONCRETE
BOTTOM

"then shovels out the moist earth below, locks the door, and goes on to "the next house. He asks no questions, and has no communication "whatever with housekeeper or servants. His work is perfectly simple, "and is performed without need for the concurrence of any one inside "the house. As the deposit which he removes is no more offensive than "so much coal-ashes, he need not work stealthily by night, like a "scavenger, and his cart in its rounds will give no offence to the public."

There is an organized Dry Earth Co. in New Haven, which is now performing service similar to that described above; and it has removed the only difficulty in the way of the introduction of the Earth System into that town. Similar arrangements are being carried into effect in several other places, and I believe that within a few years the supply of dry earth for closet use will be as universal as is now the supply of ice or coal. Wherever manure has even a moderate value, no charge should be made for renewing the earth, though of course it would be proper to charge for the first supply.

Those who are introducing Earth-Closets into their houses in a systematic way will find it desirable to connect with it a housemaid's closet, from which floor-sweepings, ashes, etc., may be thrown directly into the earth-shaft, the arrangements for removing chamber-slops (described hereafter) being in the same room.

Where it is not practicable to build closets with a drop to the cellar or down an earth-shaft, but where it is yet desirable to have more than the capacity of a commode, a fixed closet with a movable tank under the seat may be used. Figs. 7, 8, and 9 represent the appearance and construction of a closet that I have had in constant use during the past season in a close room adjoining my office. The reservoir and hopper will hold about three barrels of earth. This was filled on the 20th of May, 1869. The closet was used daily until the 20th of August, when the supply of earth was exhausted, and the tank was filled. The tank was then emptied into a large box in the same room, and the reservoir was partly filled with fresh earth. Late in October this earth was exhausted, and it was found that that which had been taken out of the tank in August was dry enough to be used again. It

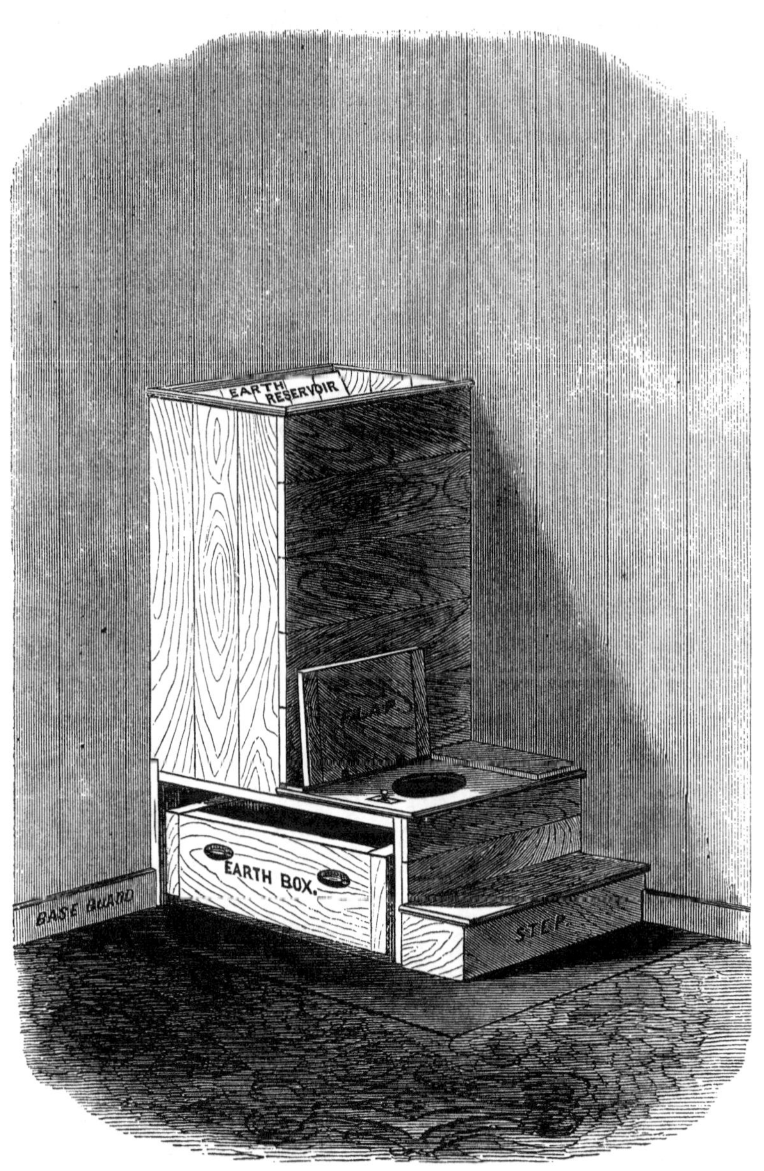

CLOSET IN CORNER OF ROOM.

was accordingly sifted and put into the hopper. There was no vestige of paper, except a little near the top of the mass, and in the whole there was not more than half a peck of solid fæces. All the rest had been completely disintegrated and absorbed by the earth. This small quantity, which probably had not decayed for want of moisture, had, when broken, the appearance and odor of rotten wood. This same lot of earth, having passed through the closet a second time, was, with its contents of excrement, removed from the tank into the box on the 24th of December, and it now has exactly the appearance and odor of any moist earth.

Since the cool weather commenced in October, this room has remained entirely unventilated, save by the occasional opening of the door leading to the office; yet it has at no time had any other odor than it would have had had it contained only a cart-load of gardener's potting-earth.

This Closet may be made larger or smaller, according to the space available for it or to the capacity required. With a vault large enough, its deposits might remain undisturbed for years, or, if necessary, they may be daily removed. Where there is only a small closet space available, the Earth-Closet may be built like an ordinary commode, raised a foot higher to admit a larger box in place of the hod, and with its back carried up a foot or two above the top of the vibrating hopper.

Figs. 10 and 11 represent a Closet with a movable tank on wheels, called a "Broadmoor Tank," which is in common use in England. This arrangement is, of course, available for a closet in the house or wood-shed, or in an outer privy.

All of these illustrations are mere suggestions for architects and builders. The plan may be varied to suit all circumstances and all tastes. The Closet may be built with oiled walnut, and highly finished, or it may be made, like one that I know of, of rough hemlock boards, in the corner of an unfinished cellar. The apparatus should be so arranged as to work freely, and to surely deposit its earth at the right point. All other conditions are unessential and may be changed at pleasure.

The foregoing directions are based on the assumption that the slight expense of procuring the patented mechanical fixtures for the Closet will not be an objection; but there are thousands of poor women and invalids in the country who cannot afford even this, yet to whom it is especially desirable to avoid the exposure that the absence of conveniences within the house makes necessary. Such conditions may be very easily met by a plan which, though less convenient, is no less effective than is the regular Moule's Closet.

Any board box of convenient size, not less than eighteen inches deep, may be fitted with a movable or hinged cover, with an ordinary finished hole. Unless the box is water-tight, its joints should be filled with putty, white-lead, tar, or pitch. Three inches of dry earth should be spread upon the bottom. At its side there should stand a box of sifted dry earth or anthracite coal-ashes, with a small tin scoop or cup. After each use of the closet, enough earth should be thrown into the box to simply cover the fæces. A pint of earth is ample for the purpose. When this box is filled, its contents may be removed with a shovel and a corn-basket, and it may be kept in the good woman's bedroom with as little offence as the stove or the chest of drawers.

Out-of-door privies, those temples of defame and graves of decency, that disfigure almost every country home in America, and raise their suggestive heads above the garden-walls of elegant town-houses, are, I believe, doomed to disappear from off the face of the earth. Twenty years ago, every back-yard in New York City was provided with one of these buildings; now, since the water-closet has come into universal use, probably there are not twenty of them to the square mile. Twenty years hence, it is to be hoped, they will become equally rare in smaller towns and in the country. That they are objectionable on the score of decency and comfort, will be confessed by all.

What is not so generally understood is their pernicious effect upon health. The influence of subterranean stores of fæcal matter in the propagation of disease has already been referred to, and will be more fully discussed hereafter; but that which produces, in the aggregate, far

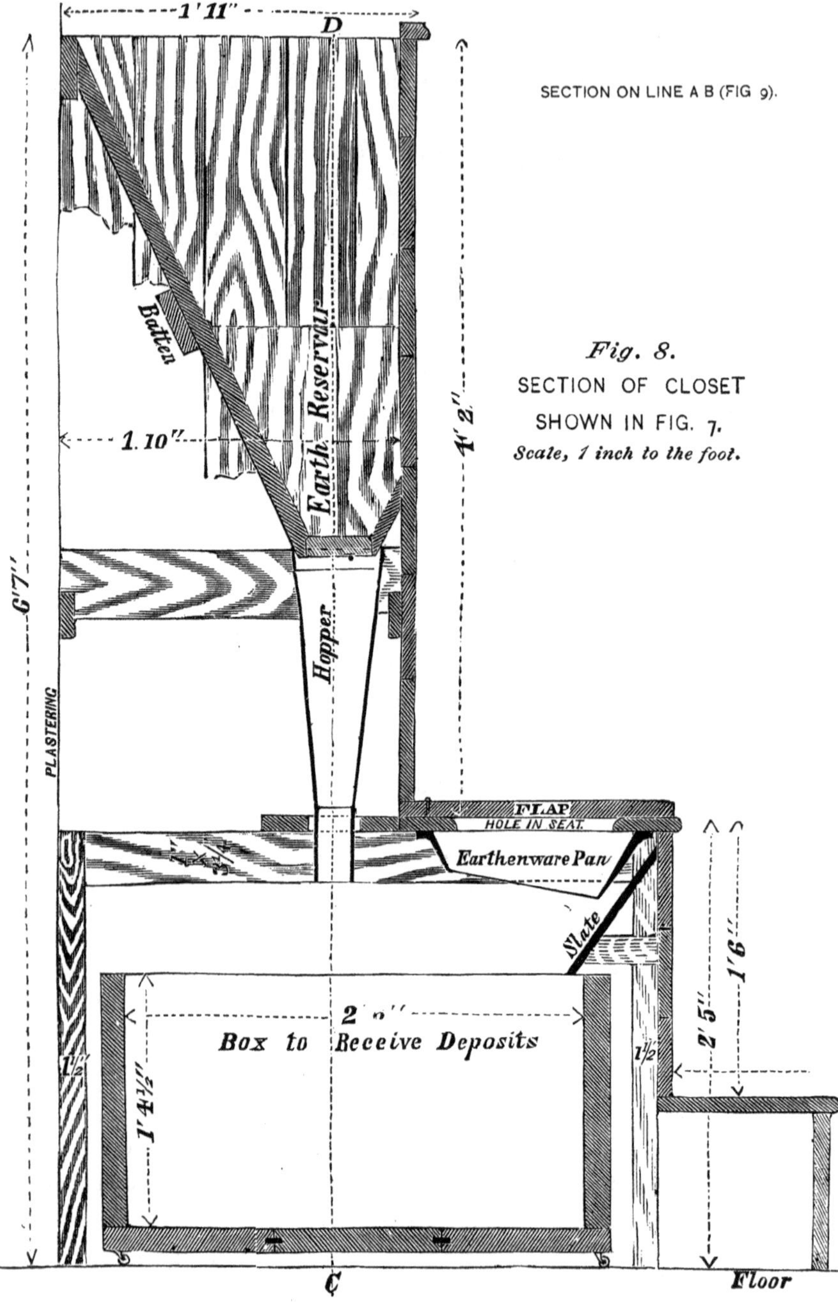

SECTION ON LINE A B (FIG 9).

Fig. 8.
SECTION OF CLOSET
SHOWN IN FIG. 7.
Scale, 1 inch to the foot.

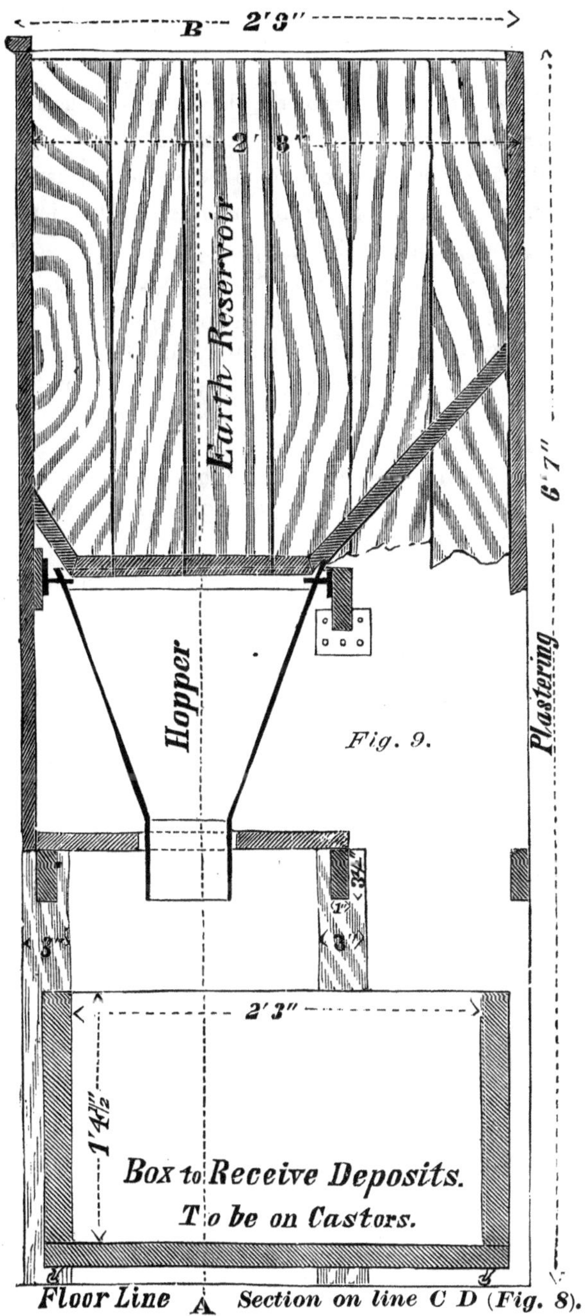

Section of Closet shown in Fig. 7.

worse results—the aggravation of the difficulties of delicate females—has attracted less attention than its importance deserves. It is universally admitted that nothing is more injurious to health than irregularity and the undue retention of the rejectamenta of the intestines. Sir James Eyre, the celebrated physician, says: *

"The bowels and the bladder, as *receiving the most hurtful excretions of our bodies*, ought not only to be emptied when they crave relief, but a wise man waits not for this; and I would implore all of either sex to remember through life that they ought to anticipate, whenever they may be able, the call to evacuate the intestinal canal. . . . The first point to be insisted on is a daily evacuation of the bowels, which can always be accomplished, the means at our command, dietetic or medicinal, being abundant, and *from this dictum no appeal whatever can be allowed.*"

But it is not necessary to quote scientific authority to prove to any person of intelligence that in prompt and regular attention to this duty lies the cardinal secret of health. We have all been reminded in our own persons that our health and efficiency, as well as our cheerfulness and good humor, depend on perfect regularity in this regard. There can be little question that the prevailing female complaints are often induced, and always intensified, by disorders of the digestive organs, and the oppression in the lower regions that neglect in this matter causes.

Admitting the justness of this view, let us see what chance a woman living in the country has to escape the direst evils that "delicate health" has in store for its victims. The privy stands, perhaps, at the bottom of the garden, fifty yards from the house, approached by a walk bordered by long grass, which is always wet except during the sunny part of the day, overhung by shrubbery and vines, which are often dripping with wet, and exposed frequently to the public gaze. In winter, snow-drifts block the way, and during rain there is no shelter from any side. The house itself is fearfully cold, if not drifted half-full with snow or flooded with rain. A woman who is comfortably housed during stormy weather will, if it is possible, postpone for days together the dreadful necessity for

* "The Stomach and its Difficulties."

exposure that such circumstances require. If the walk is exposed to a neighboring work-shop window, the visit will probably be put off until dusk. In either case, no amount of reasoning will convince a woman that it is her duty, for the sake of preventing troubles of which she is yet ignorant, to expose herself to the danger, the discomfort, and the annoyance that regularity under such circumstances implies.

I pass over now the barbarous foulness and the stifling odor of the privy-vault. It is only as an unavoidable evil that these have been tolerated; but I cannot too strongly urge attention to the point taken above, and insist on the fact that every consideration of humanity, and of the welfare not only of our own families, but of the whole community, demands a speedy reform of this abuse.

And this suggests a "woman's right," whose acquisition is more vital to her health and happiness than any that the supposed-to-be-coveted suffrage promises her; and she may, with just cause, insist that, however much she may be tyrannized over in the important matters of employment and voting, mankind has no right to hold her longer in subjection to this practical curse. It is hardly more important that she have a house to shelter her from the weather than that this incentive to a dangerous irregularity be removed.

It will hardly be believed by my more civilized readers that, over more than half of the older settled parts of the United States, even the every-way objectionable system that I have described is comparatively unknown, and that the corn-field and the thicket are the only retreat provided, while the majority of farmers' houses, even at the North, are most inadequately supplied.

In view of the foregoing facts, I make no apology for calling the attention of women themselves to this important matter, believing that they will universally concede that, however much of elegance and comfort may surround them in the appointments of their homes, their mode of life is neither decent, civilized, nor safe, unless they are provided with the conveniences that the water-closet and the earth-closet alone make possible. Being the parties most interested, it rests with them to secure the necessary relief. I should have left my task incomplete, had I

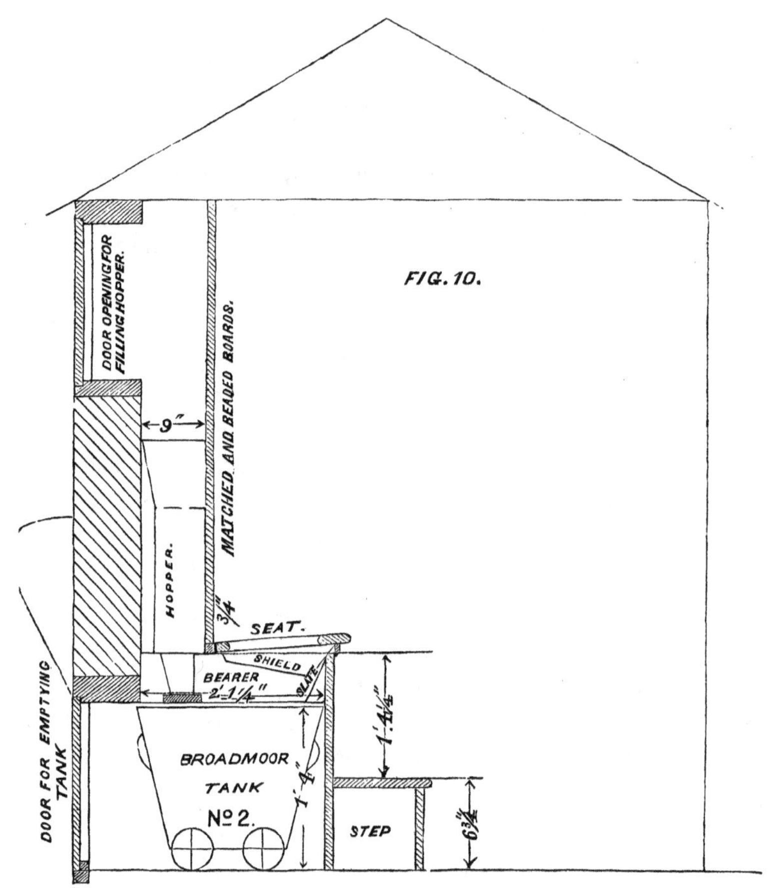

SECTION OF CLOSET WITH TANK,

TO BE SUPPLIED AND EMPTIED FROM THE REAR.

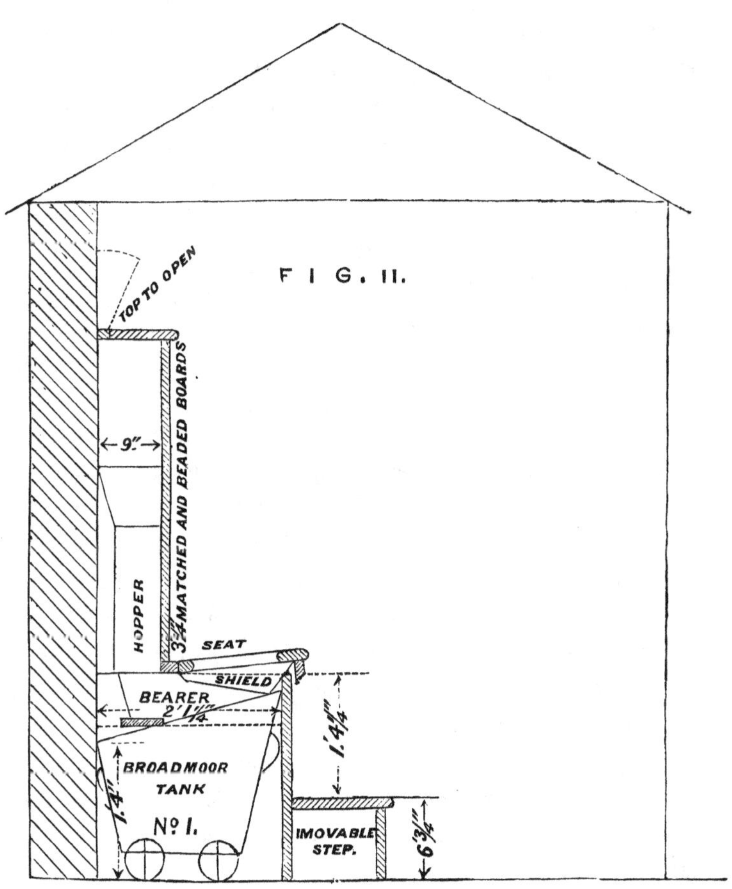

SECTION OF CLOSET WITH TANK,

TO BE SUPPLIED AND EMPTIED FROM THE INSIDE.

allowed any false notions of delicacy to deter me from making the foregoing simple but plain statement of an almost universal defect.

While believing that the detached privy building should be entirely done away with, I realize the fact that it will probably continue for some years in very general use. It becomes important, therefore, to provide for its improvement. This can be done by depriving it of its reeking vault, and converting it into an Earth-Closet, whereby its odors will be destroyed and its influence in propagating infectious diseases removed. This being done, it may be brought close to the house, perhaps connected with, or brought under, the wood-shed, thus obviating the objection of the long, exposed walk. Figs. 12 and 13 indicate a simple way in which an Earth-Closet privy may be constructed.

It will facilitate the adoption of this system to know that all of the extra appliances of a well-appointed Earth-Closet cost considerably less than an ordinary deep vault, lined with brick or stone work. The new system may be tried in a most inexpensive way, so that even the moderate outlay that the complete change requires need not be encountered until each individual has satisfied himself by his own experience of its efficiency. All that is necessary is to fill up the old vault with earth, and to provide at the side of the seat a box of dry earth or ashes, and a scoop with which to cover the fæces. This constitutes practically a complete Earth-Closet, and few who learn by its means the value of the Earth System will remain long without the greater convenience of Moule's mechanical apparatus.

For hotels, factories, railroad stations, and all other places where a number of closets are required, the expense is very much lessened by making one reservoir and one receptacle suffice for the whole series.

The plan of the soldiers' closet at Fort Adams is given in Figure 14. It would usually be necessary, at least, to add enough to the length to admit of a partition being built between the seats.

For factories having more than one floor, there are several plans by which the closets on the different stories are made to communicate with the same receptacle beneath, so that the deposits may all be removed at the ground level. The prepared earth may be taken to the different floors by the ordinary hoisting apparatus of the establishment.

COMMODES.

The form of the Earth-Closet which first commends itself to enquirers is the portable Commode, shown in Fig. 15. This is a chair, containing, in its thickened back, the vibrating hopper for holding the dry earth, and, under the seat, a hod of galvanized iron (resembling an ordinary coal-hod) for receiving the deposits. The apparatus for throwing the earth is precisely the same in all respects as that used in the large closets. I have had one of these commodes in constant use in my house for a year and a half. It usually stands in a room which connects two others that are constantly occupied. It has been used, during the whole period, three times a day on an average. The fact of its standing where it does has never prevented us from keeping the doors open into the other rooms whenever desirable. The room in which it is is used for other purposes, precisely as it would have been were the Commode not there; and, in case of sickness, it is removed into the bedroom of the invalid, its contents being carried out only when the hod is filled. Under all circumstances, it is as inoffensive and innocuous as any other piece of furniture. Keeping it in constant use, I have found it desirable to have two hods—using them alternately. With this simple precaution, and the most ordinary care to prevent the hod from becoming too full, I have found it to answer its purpose more perfectly than any water-closet I have ever seen.

If I desired to give the strongest possible proof of the entire success of the Earth System, I could not better do so than by showing this Commode in constant daily use in a close room, communicating only with two heated bedrooms, and causing no more annoyance to any member of the family than if it were a box of dry ashes. The amount of attention required is trifling. About once in four or five days the servant carries a hod of dry earth from a box in the wood-shed, and pours it into the hopper, taking the full hod out from under the seat and putting the empty one in its place. The full hod is then carried out, its contents are emptied into the manure bin, and it is hung out in

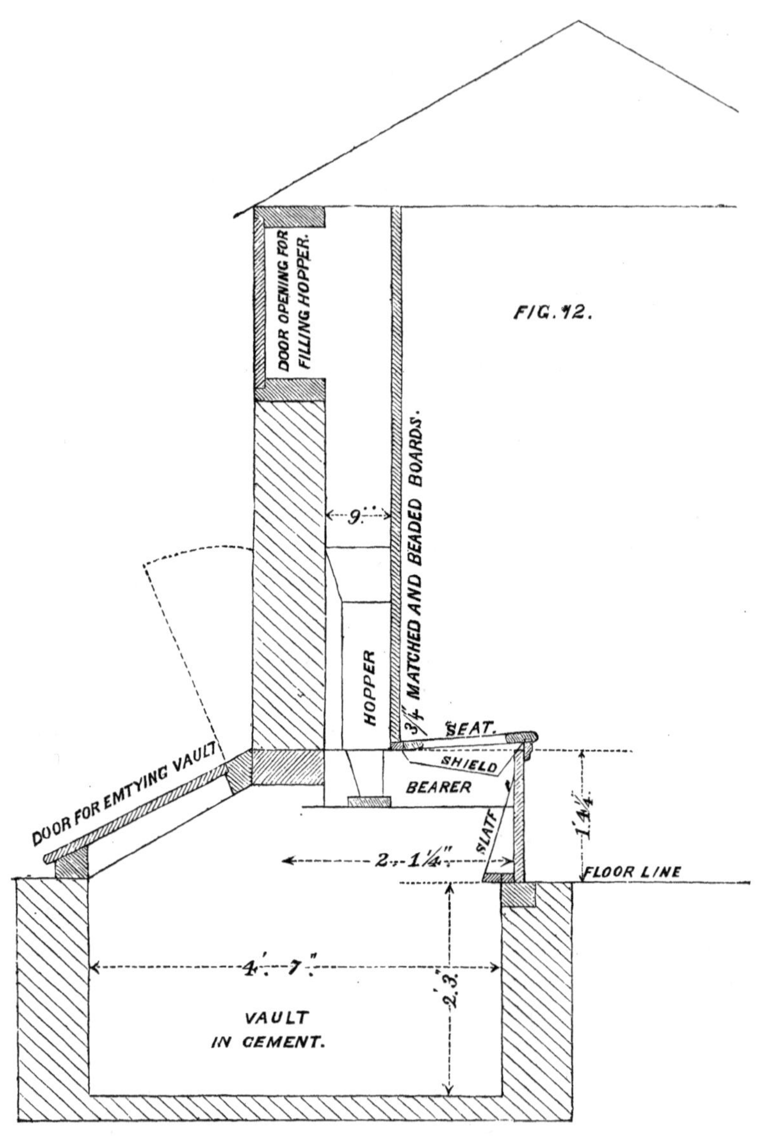

SECTION OF VAULTED PRIVY,

TO BE SUPPLIED AND EMPTIED FROM THE REAR.

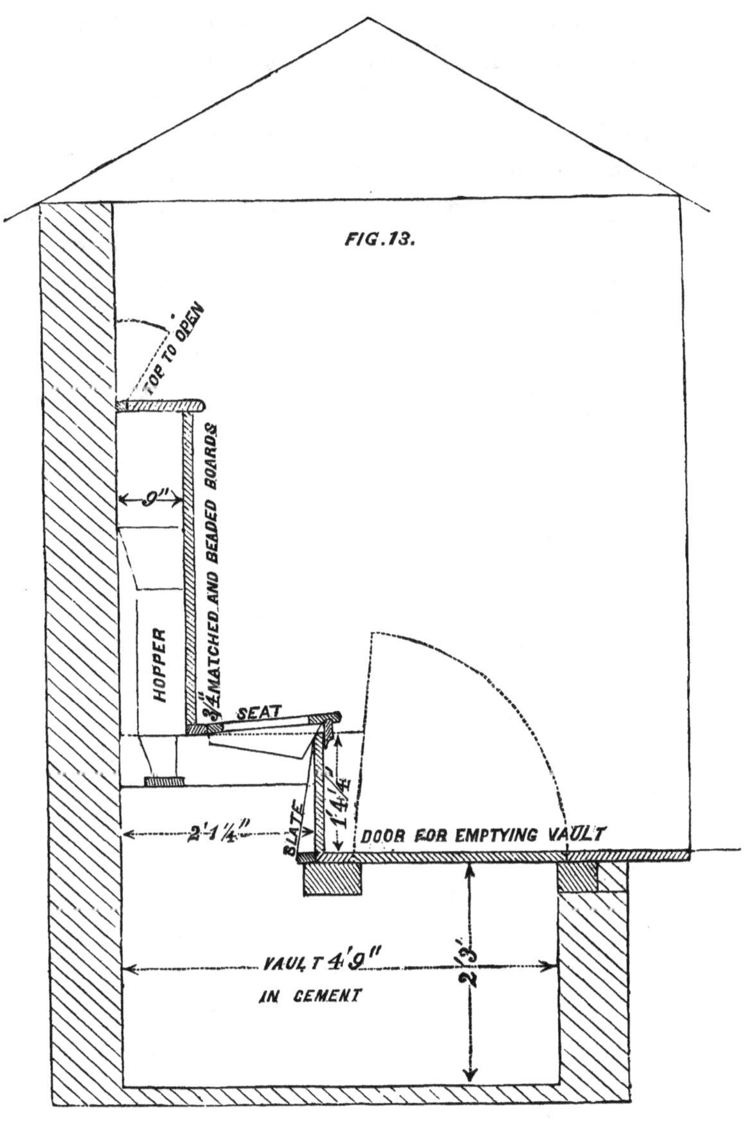

Section of Vaulted Privy showing Hopper filled and Vault emptied from Inside.

the open air, to be freshened by sun or rain until another supply of earth is required for the Commode. The labor is less than that of supplying water to the wash-stand ewers, and the annoyance is no greater than that of carrying out a hod of ashes. So invaluable has it become that it is really an indispensable part of the household appliances. As a matter of convenience, I would prefer a larger, fixed closet, in which earth enough for several months' use might be put at one time; but, as a test of the system, the Commode has better answered my purpose. Indeed, for sick-room use alone it is worth more than its cost.

BEDRIDDEN PATIENTS.

Patients who are confined absolutely to their beds are subjected to the humiliation of depending for the most intimate help on their attendants; and their recovery is, no doubt, frequently retarded by the offensive accompaniments of their care, and the depressing consciousness of the misery they inflict on others. Of course, whenever practicable, especially in prolonged cases, an arrangement similar to that of the "hospital fracture-bed" should be adopted. The mattress has a hole about ten inches in diameter, stopped by a small bit of mattress of the same thickness, covered with a piece of the ordinary sheeting. When it is in its place, the bed is smooth and comfortable. It may be easily removed from below, and a suitably arranged pan placed beneath the opening. Whether this arrangement is adopted or the ordinary bed-pan is used, perfect disinfection and deodorization may be secured by the use of dry earth, which, for this purpose, may be kept in small paper bags, holding about a pound and a half each. One of these should be emptied upon the bottom of the pan before use, and the other used to cover the exuviæ. The adoption of this simple and inexpensive device, which is within the reach of every poor woman who owns a fire-shovel, and can gain access to dry earth or dry coal-ashes, will bring untold relief to thousands of helpless invalids and their nurses, who have hitherto borne their inflictions with Christian fortitude.

In this connection, it will not be out of place to refer to the remarkable discovery of Dr. Hewson concerning the healing effect of dry earth when applied to open wounds. I had the good fortune to attend a

FLOOR
SEAT
1'6"
2'
HOPPER
STEPS
A
B
C
D
PLAN OF EARTH CLOSETS
SOLDIERS'
EARTH-CLOSETS
AT
FORT ADAMS.
NEWPORT, R.I.
EARTH RESERVOIR
HOPPER
2'
1'6"
8'2"
SILL
VAULT
6'
2'
8"
SECTION ON A.B.
EARTH RESERVOIR
FLAP
1'5"
2'11"
FLOOR JOIST
VAULT
4"4"
SECTION ON C.D

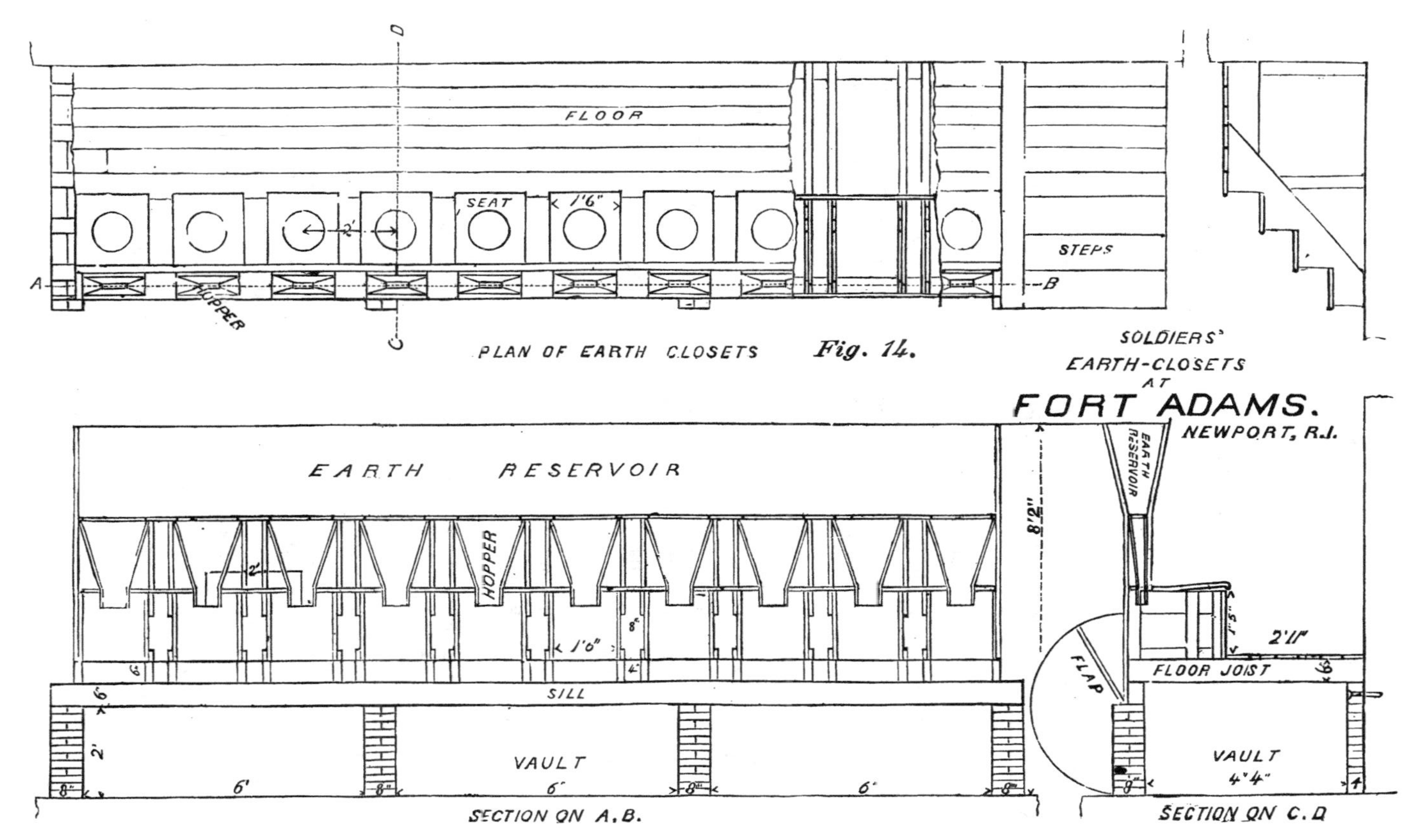

Fig. 14.

morning dressing of the surgical cases in the Pennsylvania Hospital, and sent the following communication to the New York *Evening Post:*

"THE EARTH-CLOSET, AND THE TREATMENT OF WOUNDS.

"One of the experimental Commodes, sent out by the Earth-Closet "Company of Hartford, was placed at the disposal of Dr. Addinell Hew- "son, of the Pennsylvania Hospital (in Philadelphia). Its introduction "into the surgical ward, where it has been for two weeks in constant use "by about twenty patients, and has been subjected to the severest test "possible, has been so entirely satisfactory that it is proposed to substi- "tute Earth-Closets for water-closets wherever these exist in the institu- "tion.

"At the time of its introduction, there was lying in the ward a "patient suffering from a very severe compound fracture of the lower "leg. The wound was in an unhealthy condition, and its exudations, "amounting to a pint in twenty-four hours, were so offensive as to cause "a sickening, even dangerous, stench, that the excellent ventilation of the "ward and the usual disinfectants were hardly able even to mitigate. It "occurred to Dr. Hewson to test the power of dry earth to absorb this "odor, as it had that of excrement. The effect was magical. Not only "was the offensiveness entirely overcome, but the effect on the character "of the wound itself was such as no previous treatment had been able to "compass. The suppuration was, within a few days, so reduced that "the daily dressing of a single half pint of earth was not even saturat- "ed; the edges of the flesh wound lost their inflamed character; the "intense pain of the sore was entirely relieved, and a healthy granu- "lation has ensued.

"Such an indication of a newly-found healing-agent was not dis- "regarded.

"On Monday last, being in Philadelphia, I was invited to attend "the morning dressing of the earth-treated wounds. This is what "I saw:

"*First.* Two patients, suffering from serious varicose ulcers, after "prolonged suffering, and with little relief from the usual treatment, "have ceased to be offensive to their wardmates; they find their sores "growing daily smaller; all pain and inflammation have left them; and "they feel the certainty of an early cure.

"*Second.* A railroad brakeman, whose hand was, a year and a "half ago, crushed between the coupling-heads of two cars, and who "has never been free from pain, and seldom from intense pain; whose

THE MECHANICAL PARTS OF THE COMMODE.

The same Fixtures are used in Closets.

Fig. 15.

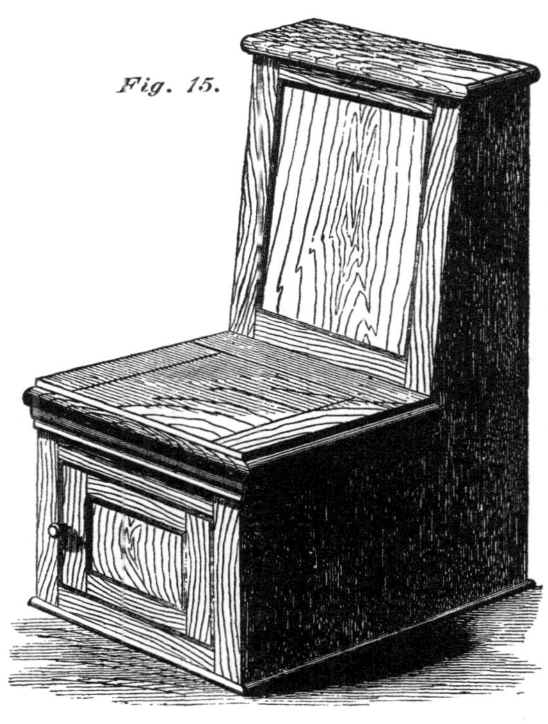

THE COMMODE.

" hand, from the wrist to the knuckles, was a festering mass of carious " bones and inflamed flesh, and whose system had been so reduced " that he could not have survived the amputation, which alone can en- " tirely relieve him, is now happy in freedom from pain. His flesh- " wound has taken on a healthy character, and his strength is fast return- " ing. He even hopes to save his hand, but the long-continued decay " of the bone makes this impossible.

" *Third.* Another brakeman, suffering from a precisely similar " injury, in no respect less serious, but received within a few days, was " immediately treated with dry earth. Its constant application has en- " tirely prevented inflammation, and a healthy healing of the flesh and " knitting of the bone will soon return him to his duties with two useful " hands.

" *Fourth.* A farm laborer, on Friday last, had three of his fingers " nearly cut off and fearfully torn by a horse-power hay-cutter. Since " the first application of the dry earth (a few hours after the accident) " he has been free from pain, and he will save his hand.

" *Fifth.* On Saturday last, a laborer, engaged in breaking up con- " demned shells, exploded one that was charged. The powder burned " his face and arms, and (seriously) one of his knees, which was struck " by a fragment of the iron that completely shattered the knee-pan. " His burns and the fracture were immediately dressed with dry earth, " and the freedom from pain and the absence of inflammation have been " as marked in this case as in the others. Without this dressing the " knee-joint must inevitably have become involved, and the leg must " have been lost. Now the wound is evidently healing, and (although " it is too early to speak positively) there is every reason to hope that " the only result of the injury will be a stiff knee.

" *Sixth.* Within a few days a woman was brought to the hospital, " with her neck and a large part of her body very severely and danger- " ously burned. That she could escape long weeks of agony was be- " yond hope. Yet on Monday her eye was clear and calm, and her " voice was strong; but when the doctor asked her how she felt, she " said she was a great deal better, and that she had no pain.

" *Seventh.* Last Wednesday, an entire breast was removed for " cancer, and the wound was dressed with dry earth. It is now healing " rapidly. There has been no inflammation and no suppuration; and " this woman, too—calm and happy-looking, with a healthy color and " a steady voice—spoke far more than her cheerful words in thankful- " ness for her relief.

"Surely, with our gratitude to the Vicar of Fordington, who has "conferred the greatest benefit on the human race that it has ever been "given to one person to accomplish, we must unite our thanks to the "senior surgeon of the Pennsylvania Hospital for thus applying the "principles of his invention to the saving of life and limb, and to the "alleviation of unspeakable suffering.

"And the end, I trust, is not yet. It seems inevitable that the "pustules of small-pox must give up their pain and their offensiveness "at this magic touch of mother earth; and if it is true that this conta-"gion spreads from its exudations, may we not hope that Dr. Hewson "has bound its feet, as Mr. Moule has those of cholera?"

Nearly a year has passed since this discovery was made, and Dr. Hewson has continued his investigations most zealously. I have been enabled to examine the evidence of almost universal success with which his practice has been attended, which he is now preparing for publication.

My communication to the New York *Post* brought many letters from suffering people and their friends in all parts of the country; and from subsequent correspondence I am glad to have learned that much good has resulted. I *know* that one life has been saved by Dr. Hewson's discovery (and I believe that at least one other has been) within my own observation.

The prophecy concerning small-pox has been fulfilled in San Francisco, as is shown by the following extract from the *Pacific Medical and Surgical Journal*, November, 1869, from a report of "Observations on "the late Epidemic Small-pox," by Thomas M. Logan, M.D., Secretary of the Board of Health, and late Physician to the Small-pox Hospital, Sacramento:

"Another improvement in the hospital system is found in the dry-"earth treatment. Not only did it prove the best deodorizer, but at "the magic touch of mother earth the pustules and festering sores of "small-pox gave up their pain and offensiveness, healing up kindly "without any other dressing."

HOUSE SLOPS.

In considering the question of Earth Sewage as a complete substitute for the water system, a serious question arose concerning the disposition of the liquid wastes of sleeping-rooms and kitchen. Obviously the adoption of the Earth-Closet as a universal system, with the entire exclusion not only of the common privy and water-closet, but of the cess-pools and public sewers (as a means for removing filth), could not be effected unless some sufficient means were provided for the removal of the liquid wastes of the house, and for a long time this question seemed to doom the Earth-Closet to an accessory position.

For example, the authorities of a growing town, contemplating the adoption of some system for the removal of its domestic wastes, in examining the operation of earth-sewage, find that, although for a single purpose the Earth-Closet is admirably suited to their wants, the entire absence of a provision for removing all manner of *house-slops* leaves it insufficient for their purpose, and they turn to the regular water-supply and street-sewer plan that is in common use.

Little by little, by experiments here and in England, this want has been provided for, and the system of Earth-Sewage may now be considered complete.

The different cases to be considered are the following :

1. The isolated country-house, which has hitherto depended entirely upon cess-pools, but which has a garden or lawn adjoining it.

2. The town-house, which has very little land, and, at the same time, has no communication with any public sewer or drain.

3. The city-house, that has practically no land about it, but adjoins a public sewer or water-conduit.

1. Country-houses, with vegetable gardens, flower borders, shrubbery, fruit-trees, or grape-vines, should adopt the percolating-drain system (which is illustrated in Fig. 16), which is a representation of the device by which the slops of my own kitchen are disposed of. The drain, from the corner of the house to the cistern, is made of three-inch vitrified pipes, with cemented joints, so that there can be no escape of moisture anywhere between the house and the cistern. This latter is, in my case, a kerosene barrel, sunk in the ground until its open top is level with the surface. The cemented pipe enters it about ten inches below

the top. From the points *a* and *b*, about twelve inches below the top of the barrel, holes are made to receive common three-inch land-drain tiles. Each of these side-drains extends eight feet from the barrel. Connected with them by the use of Boynton's curves and junction pieces, the four drains, *c*, *d*, *e*, and *f*, extend across the garden, a distance of about fifty feet, running in parallel lines six feet apart. The joints of these drains and of the side-drains, *a* and *b*, are connected only with open collars, leaving room for the free percolation of water through them. The barrel itself is provided with a wire-cloth screen, reaching from the top to the bottom, and separating the side of the barrel into which the house-drain empties from that out of which the other drains lead. This holds back the coarser matters of the drainage, which, by their decomposition, make a thick scum on the top of the liquid, which I found sufficient to choke up the screens over the outlet-pipes which I at first adopted. The vertical screen answers its purpose perfectly. The barrel itself—that part of it lying below the level of the drains—forms a pool for subsidence, corresponding with the silt-basin in land drainage. The pipes are laid twelve inches, or less, below the surface of the ground. The liquid which enters them from the barrel is of a milky color, but seems to be free from any substance that can choke them up. The liquid leaking out through the joints is absorbed by the soil, and adds greatly to its fertility, and, possibly, gives it in dry weather an appreciable amount of moisture at a point where plants can make use of it. I have had this system in operation now about six months. It is thus far perfectly satisfactory, and I see no reason why it should not permanently continue so. It is possible that in time the joints may become choked and prevent the percolation of the water. Should this occur, it will not require more than a half-day's work to take the pipes all up, clean them, and relay them.

If I were to repeat this operation, I should lay the pipes within eight inches of the surface, and probably a more perfect manuring would be effected if they were only three feet apart instead of six feet.

I have been enabled to do away entirely with an offensive cesspool that stood within twenty feet of the house, and have a substitute

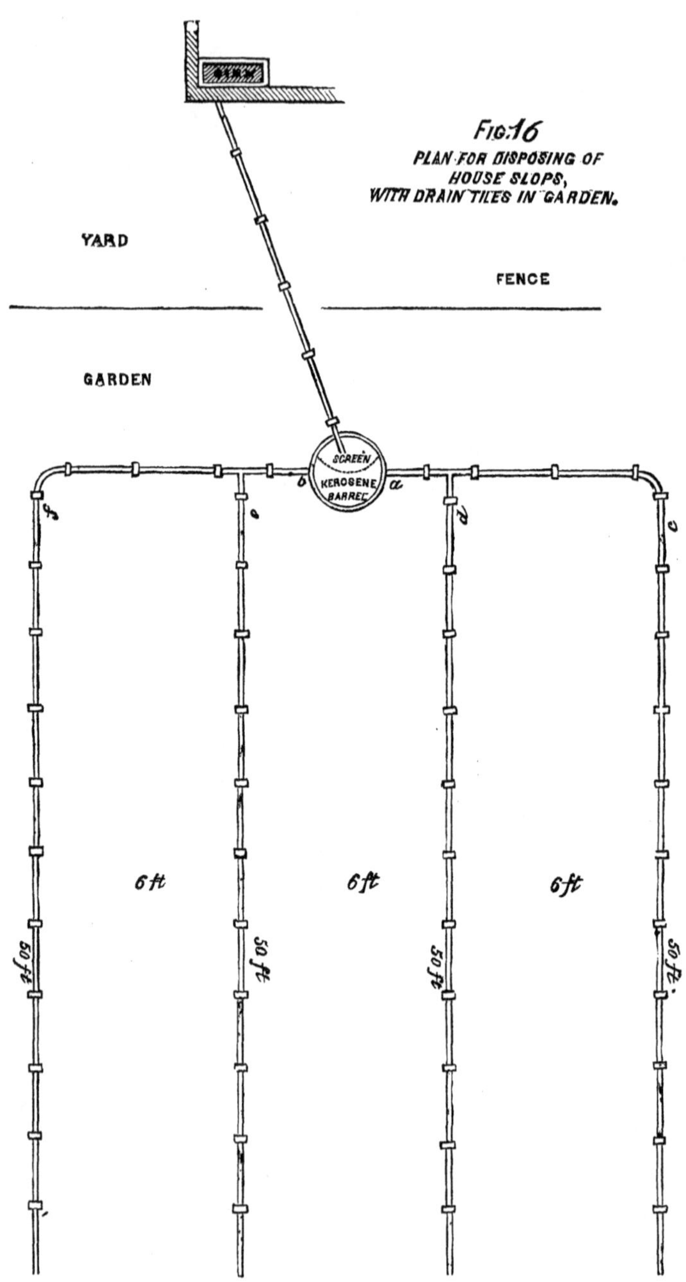

FIG. 16
PLAN FOR DISPOSING OF HOUSE SLOPS, WITH DRAIN TILES IN GARDEN.

from which it is impossible to detect the slightest odor, even in midsummer.

In a colder climate it might be necessary to cover the ground with leaves or straw directly over the pipes, to protect them from frost.

The cost of this arrangement, in my case, has been as follows:

40 feet 3-inch vitrified pipe	$6 80
16 " 3-inch drain-pipe	64
200 " 1½ " " with collars . . .	6 00
1 kerosene barrel	1 00
Labor and cement	2 50
Total	$16 94

I have no doubt that the value of the manure will exceed this amount every year.

The suggestion for this work I found in the following, which is extracted from the advertising circular of Moule's Patent Earth-Closet Company in London:

"HOUSE SLOPS, ETC.

"Where there is a garden, the house-slops and sink-water may, "in most cases, be made of great value, and removed from the house "without the least annoyance. The only requirement is that there shall "be a gradual incline from the house to the garden. Let all the slops "fall into a trapped sink, the drain from which to the garden should "be of glazed socket pipes, well jointed, and emptying itself into a "small tank, eighteen inches deep, about one foot wide, and of such "length as may be necessary. The surplus rain-water from the roof "may also enter this. Out of this tank, lay three-inch common drain-"pipes, eight feet apart, and twelve inches below the surface. Lay "mortar at top and bottom of the joint, leaving the sides open. If "these pipes are extended to a considerable length, small tanks, about "one foot square and eighteen inches deep, must be sunk at about "every twenty or forty feet, to allow for subsidence. These can easily "be emptied as often as required; and the deposit may be either "mixed with dry earth or be dug in at once as a manure. The liquid "oozes into the cultivated soil; and the result is something fabulous. "This simple plan will effectually deal with the slops; there is no smell,

" no possibility of any foul gas to poison the atmosphere, and with this, " and the produce of the Earth-Closet, any ground may be productive " and profitable.

" The two following facts will illustrate the value of this system of " dealing with house-slops, etc.

" On a wall fifty-five feet in length and sixteen feet high a vine " grows. A three-inch pipe runs parallel with this at a distance of six " feet from it for the entire length; the slops flow through this pipe as " above described. On this vine, year after year, had been grown four " hundred well-ripened bunches of grapes, some of the bunches weigh- " ing three-quarters of a pound. During a period of four years, for a " certain purpose, the supply was cut off. To the surprise of the gar- " dener, scarcely any grapes during those years appeared; but afterwards " the supply was restored, and the consequence was an abundant crop; " the wood grew fully sixteen feet, of good size and well ripened.

" The other case was as follows:

" Pipes were laid below two square yards of earth, twelve inches " beneath the surface, which were fed with the slops through an upright " pipe, about one large watering-potful daily. In the month of Novem- " ber, three roots of Tartarian oats were planted in this piece of ground. " The stalks attained one inch and a quarter in circumference; the " leaves measured an inch across.

" Several of the ears were twenty-six inches long, and when the " crop was gathered eight hundred grains were rubbed out of one ear. " The whole weight of corn from those plants was three-quarters of a " pound. Twelve of these grains were put into the same piece of " ground the following year: from these was grown one pound and " three-quarters of seed. In fact, in a garden of twenty perches, by the " use of both solid and liquid manure from one house, three crops were " grown in the year, the value of which at market price would be twen- " ty pounds.

" In a garden in which this plan has been adopted for eight or ten " years, the pipes were recently taken up in order to see how far they " might have been filled with the mud of subsidence. After so long " use, very little subsidence was found, and none to obstruct the " working of the system, excepting where, in one or two places, the bad " laying of the pipes caused some obstruction. There was nothing " which might not at any time be remedied in half an hour.

" It will be easily seen that this mode of removing sink-water and " slops can be applied to towns or districts of towns. Whilst the appli-

" cation of liquid sewage, in the ordinary sense of that expression, to the " purposes of irrigation will be generally impossible, either from the " want of proper land or proper fall, or the extravagant cost of pump- " ing, or the difficulty of irrigating during frost or during harvest, this " small portion of the refuse-matter of towns, rendered more easy of dis- " tribution by the admixture of rain-water, can be pumped to any " height, even to land above the town, at all seasons and under all cir- " cumstances. During the hard frost of 1867, the sub-irrigation in the " garden above mentioned has continued without the slightest interrup- " tion."

2. Town-houses, which have too little land, or about which the soil is too sandy for the foregoing system to be adopted, may be relieved of their liquid wastes by filtering them through earth in a large cask or other vessel.

This plan I have had in operation for more than a year; first, during the winter of 1868–69, under the kitchen sink of my gardener's house, there being five persons in the family. A single charge of earth lasted for four months. At the end of that time, the water oozing from the bottom of the hogshead was slightly discolored, and its contents were required to be renewed. Frost was excluded by filling the upper six inches of the barrel with horse manure. This allowed the infiltration of the liquid even in the coldest weather. When the contents of the cask were removed, they were spread upon one of two parallel cold frames, intended for lettuce. The corresponding frame received $20 worth (2½ cords) of livery-stable manure. The land had not previously been manured for a long time. The crop grown by the cask-manure was much the more luxuriant and valuable of the two.

This experiment having proved so successful, when I arranged for the disposal of my kitchen-drain as above described, I prepared a similar cask in my own garden to receive the chamber-slops of the house. This cask, with a leaky bottom, stands on the top of the ground, and is filled three-fourths full with earth (the unprepared surface soil of the garden). It is covered with a round cover of matched boards, well battened together, and provided with a funnel similar to the one shown in Fig. 17, having a closely fitting flat cover, which is ordinarily kept closed. This hogshead was put in use in August. Before very long the earth, which contains a good deal of clay, was so puddled as to prevent the entrance of the liquids, or, at least, admitted them very slowly, so that there was usually water standing in the funnel. This was remedied for a time by filling in with coal-ashes on top of the earth. How long this would have lasted in warm weather, I cannot say. It worked well until it froze. I then had all of the ashes and a little of the earth removed, and packed the barrel full with very coarse stable-manure, fully three-fourths straw. The funnel was also half-filled with the same material. This was about the middle of November, and, as I write, two months later, the operation is perfect—the entire up-stairs waste of the establishment being completely disposed of, and there being as yet no indication that anything but clear water (plenty of that) has escaped at the bottom.

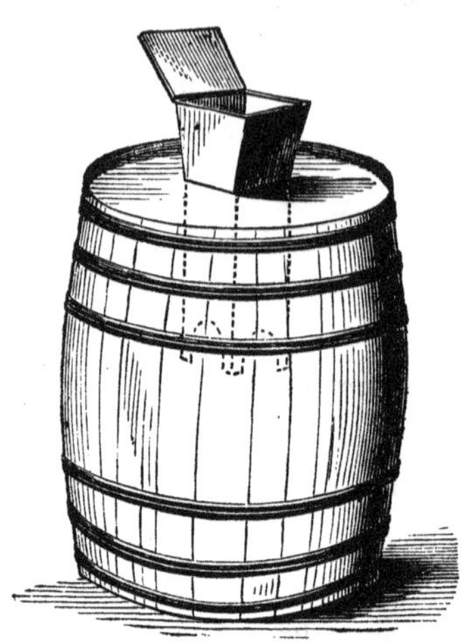

Fig. 17.

The cost of such an apparatus as this is too trifling to be considered, in view of its great value as a means of ridding ourselves of one of the worst pests of ordinary village housekeeping. The same cask may receive both the up-stairs and down-stairs wastes, just as the same system of drains might do.

Where there is even a small garden or a single grape arbor, I believe that the drain method is the best. The other would be generally practicable in towns with the co-operation of farmers and gardeners. The cask, with its cover and funnel, being provided, any farmer or gardener would gladly supply it with earth, and replenish it two or three times a year, for the sake of the manure.

3. Where sewers are already established in towns, and it is decided no longer to admit the washings of water-closets, or where a clear-water drainage only is provided for, such householders as have not sufficient land to adopt the drain-tile sewage plan will require to filter their house-liquids before sending them to the public conduits.

It is proposed, in the Riverside plan previously alluded to, to allow no connection to be made with the public drains, except through pipes so small that they would be obstructed by the subsidence from even semi-fluid house-wastes. It will be necessary, therefore, to adopt one of two plans:

First. To receive all of the house drainage into a subsidence-pool or silt-basin, having at least the capacity of a barrel. The drain from the house should enter this near the top, and the outlet drain should be at about the same level, so that the lower part of the barrel may remain entirely filled, and that its contents may not be unduly disturbed by the liquids running into it. Between the inlet and the outlet drains there should be a vertical wire-cloth screen, as previously described. Of course this vessel should be closely covered. This plan is subject to the objections that it allows the manurial constituents of the liquids to pass off in solution, and that it contaminates the waters of the stream into which the sewer discharges.

Second. Or, which is very much better, to filter all of the house liquids through a mass of charcoal or mixed charcoal and gravel. For this purpose, there will be required a somewhat larger cask or other suitable receptacle, filled with the filtering material, and so protected in winter that its contents cannot be frozen. The foul liquids received at the top of the cask will pass off through a drain at its bottom, deprived of their impurity. There should be some access for air at the top of the cask. This will follow the subsidence of the liquid, and assist in destroying the organic deposits.

Where it is not thought necessary to do more than prevent the entrance of semi-solid matters into the drain, it will be sufficient to provide the sinks and funnels into which the liquids are poured, in the house, with suitable strainers. As it is especially desirable to obviate the necessity for carrying waste water from the upper floors of the house, there should be, in connection with the Earth-Closet, a funnel or sink into which they may be poured. The best form, as requiring the least space, will be an earthen-ware funnel, about twelve inches in diameter at its top, discharging into a two-inch or three-inch vitrified pipe, with cemented joints. This pipe may, at its lower end, communicate with a system of drain-tiles in the garden, with a cask of earth or of charcoal, or directly with the public drain.

The earthen-ware funnel should contain a funnel-shaped strainer of galvanized wire-cloth, having two convenient handles (on opposite sides). This strainer should be somewhat smaller than the earthen-ware funnel, except at its rim, and it would be safer to have a second strainer not movable below it. The funnel-shaped strainer will retain hair, paper, and other substances which might choke the drain; and when these have accumulated so as to retard the flow of the liquids, it may be lifted out of the funnel by its handles, and emptied down the earth-shaft adjoining.

I have not seen all of the foregoing systems of drainage in operation, but I have experimented sufficiently on the subject to be confident that they are entirely practicable, and that they include provisions suited to all ordinary cases.

THE MANURE QUESTION.

IT is a very difficult matter to fix the value of any animal manure, except by accurate analysis of each separate sample. Opinions as to the value of human excrement vary widely according to the standard of comparison taken. It is a singular fact (which does not obtain with reference to most other manures) that the valuation of human excrement made by chemists is very much less than that of the practical farmer. For instance, in England, where the value of the mineral constituents of the material seems to be entirely disregarded, it is usual to measure the value solely by the amount of *ammonia* that may be produced from it; those parts of night-soil which are the key to the lasting fertility of the land are not taken into the account, and ammonia alone (which, although a most valuable and efficient aid to the farmer, counts as nothing in giving permanent fertility) is considered. By this estimate, the value of human excrement is fixed at about $2 for each individual, an amount which any market-gardener or farmer, who depends mainly on night-soil as a source of manure, would consider absurdly low. Professor Johnson has told us that, years ago, in the days of low prices, the excrement of a man was considered in Flanders to be worth $9 a year.

In this connection, I reproduce a portion of an article written for Judd's *Agricultural Annual* of 1868:*

" The average population of New York City—including its temporary visitors—is probably not less than 1,000,000. This population consumes food equivalent to at least 30,000,000 bushels of corn in a

* "Sewers and Earth-Closets, and their Relation to Agriculture."

year. Excepting the small proportion that is stored up in the bodies of the growing young, which is fully offset by that contained in the bodies of the dead, the constituents of the food are returned to the air by the lungs and skin, or are voided as excrement. That which goes to the air was originally taken from the air by vegetation, and will be so taken again. Here is no waste. The excrement contains all that was furnished by the mineral elements of the soil on which the food was produced. This all passes into the sewers, and is washed into the sea. Its loss, to the present generation, is complete.

"In the present half-developed condition of the world, there is no help for this. The first duty in all towns is to remove from the vicinity of habitations all matters which, by their decomposition, would tend to produce disease. The question of health is, of course, of the first importance, and that of economy must follow it; but it should follow closely, and perfect civilization must await its solution.

"Thirty million bushels of corn contain, among other minerals, nearly seven thousand tons of phosphoric acid, and this amount is annually lost in the wasted night-soil of New York City.*

"Practically, the human excrement of the whole country is nearly all so disposed of as to be lost to the soil. The present population of the United States is not far from 35,000,000. On the basis of the above calculation, their annual food contains over 200,000 tons of phosphoric acid, being about the amount contained in 900,000 tons of bones, which, at the price of the best flour of bone (for manure), would be worth over $50,000,000. It would be a moderate estimate to say that the other constituents of food found in night-soil are of at least equal value with the other constituents of the bone, and to assume $50,000,000 as the money value of the wasted night-soil of the United States.

"In another view, the importance of this waste cannot be estimated in money. Money values apply, rather, to the products of labor, and to the exchange of these products. The waste of fertilizing matters reaches farther than the destruction or exchange of products—it lessens the ability to produce.

"If mill-streams were failing year by year, and steam were yearly

* Other mineral constituents of food—important ones, too—are washed away in even greater quantities through the same channels; but this element is the best for illustration, because its effect in manure is the most striking, even so small a dressing as twenty pounds per acre producing a marked effect on all cereal crops. Ammonia, too, which is so important that it is usual in England to estimate the value of manure in exact proportion to its supply of this element, is largely yielded by human excrement.

losing force, and the ability of men to labor were yearly growing less, the doom of our prosperity would not be more plainly written than if the slow but certain impoverishment of our soil were sure to continue.

"Fortunately, it will not continue always. So long as there are virgin soils, this side of the Pacific, which our people can ravage at will, thoughtless earth-robbers will move West and 'till' them. But the good time is coming, when (as now in China and in Japan) men must accept the fact that the soil is not a warehouse to be plundered —only a factory to be worked. Then they will save their raw material, instead of wasting it; and, aided by nature's wonderful loom, will weave, over and over again, the fabric by which we live and prosper. Men will build up as fast as men destroy, old matters will be reproduced in new forms, and, as the decaying forests feed the growing wood, so will all consumed food yield food again.

"The stupendous sewers which have just been completed in London at a cost of $20,000,000, and which challenge admiration as monuments of engineering achievement, are a great blessing to that filth-accursed town, and, in the absence of anything better, they might, with advantage, be imitated elsewhere. They have had an excellent effect on the health of the population, by removing a prolific cause of typhoid fever and other fatal diseases. As affording needed relief from malaria, they are of immense importance. Still, they are a great (although necessary) evil, inasmuch as they wash into the sea the manurial products of 3,000,000 people, to supply whom with food requires the importation of immense quantities of grain and manure.

"The wheat market of one-half the world is regulated by the demand in England. She draws food from the Black Sea and from California; she uses most of the guano of the Pacific islands; she even ransacks the battle-fields of Europe for human bones, from which to make fresh bones for her people; and, in spite of all this, her food is scarce and high, and bread-riots break out in her towns.

"An earnest effort is now being made to use the matters discharged through these sewers for the fertilizing of the lands toward the eastern coast. For this purpose, it is intended to build a sewer, forty miles long and nine and a half feet in diameter, which, with the incidental expenses of its construction and management, will cost about $10,000,000. The sewage company have a farm at Barking, on which they have experimented very successfully, one acre of their irrigated meadows having produced nine tons of Italian rye grass in twenty-two days, and fifty tons during the past season up to August

15, with a prospect that the yield for the whole season will be, at least, seventy tons from a single acre.

"The system of sewage irrigation has earnest adherents, and equally earnest opposers. It does seem a pity that, for every pound of excrement that is given to the land, three or four hundred pounds of water must go with it; and it is probable that such highly diluted manure can be used with advantage only on grass crops. It is further asserted that, as the best results can be obtained only by the application of from 6,000 to 10,000 tons of the liquid per acre, the cost of the process must prevent its general adoption. However, the scheme is about to be thoroughly tested, and it is to be hoped that its success will be such as to secure a return to the soil of a vast amount of valuable matter which, hitherto, has been worse than thrown away.

"The many attempts that have been made to extract the fertilizing parts of the sewage from the deluge of water with which they are diluted, have entirely failed of their object. If, as now seems probable, the best and cheapest way to remove waste matters from large towns is by dilution in large quantities of water, the efforts of agriculturists must be directed to the best means of making use of the mixture."

Since this paper was written, a further investigation of the subject has forced me to the conclusion that the value of night-soil is very much greater than I at that time placed it, and I believe that I am not unwarranted in saying that the value of the entire product of a household, including chamber, kitchen, and laundry wastes, when utilized by means of the Earth System, is worth $10 for each individual of the family.

My own family numbers five persons; every particle of the waste is utilized in the best manner, and I am confident that I shall receive, from the accumulation of the year, more benefit from the product than I would from $50 worth of any manure that I could purchase. Wherever I have used either the earth from the Closet or the contents of my filtering-casks, the effect has been obviously much greater than it would have been from the use of the raw material alone. A portion of the improvement, no doubt, is due to the more even distribution that the increased bulk makes possible; but I am inclined to attach much greater importance to a suggestion contained in an article prepared by Colonel Weld for the *Agricultural Annual* for 1870. He says:

" Most soils contain a much larger quantity of substances required " by the plant than would be available in several years' cropping. These " are gradually rendered soluble and fit for plant-food by weathering " year by year. The result of mingling a soil with manure which is un- " dergoing active fermentation is to cause decomposition to go on in it " more rapidly, and so it is certain that a part of the benefit arising from " the use of soil as an absorbent in stables is that a larger supply of " plant-food is prepared from the soil and distributed with the ma- " nure."

Of course this introduces an element of uncertainty into the calculation, as it is not likely that any two soils would yield exactly the same fertilizing value to the action of the manure; but it is undoubtedly true that any earth not positively barren will be very beneficially affected by the active decomposition of fæces and urine within its mass.

The same article contains the following lucid statement of the effect of earth on decomposing organic matter:

" The Earth-Closet depends for its working upon the deodorizing " and absorbing qualities of dry earth. The earth absorbs moisture " because it is dry; it absorbs odors, both on account of its chemical " nature and the mechanical arrangement of its particles. Earth is " sometimes considered as antiseptic, because it so thoroughly destroys " some of the products of decay, especially evil odors; but it really pro " motes decay very energetically. If we lift a piece of cloth, a part of " which has been buried by accident for a few days or weeks, we find " the part under the earth greatly injured, or entirely rotten, from the " contact of earth and moisture. Very dry earth is somewhat antiseptic " on account of its dryness.

" The disorganization or decay which earth promotes does not " affect living organisms of either plants or animals. Hence, seeds, " roots, bulbs, insect life, and the eggs of many birds, reptiles, and in- " sects, are preserved, if buried in earth of natural dryness, so long as " life remains.

" The purifying and deodorizing properties of the soil are familiar " to almost every farmer boy in the country. A very slight burying " prevents the odor of a decaying carcass being noticeable; a thin cover- " ing of earth suffices to suppress the odors of a fresh manure heap; and " the most disgusting of all common smells, that of the skunk, may be

" entirely removed from articles of clothing, or other things contaminat-
" ed by it, by burying them in the ground a few weeks (of course, ab-
" solute contact of the earth with the garments should be prevented, or
" they would be rendered useless through decay)."

The manner in which the closet manure should be prepared for use will be described in connection with the question of earth supply and removal.

There is one consideration connected with this branch of the subject which is of even greater importance than the mere money value of the single application of the manure. Our present system is one of constant waste. We draw from the soil a certain amount of plant-food with every crop that we grow. In so far as the crop is consumed by man, this plant-food is practically wasted. In the next crop that the land produces, fresh elements are required, and these, in their turn, are thrown away. And so we go on, year after year, always drawing out more than we put back, to the extent of almost the entire food of our population. Of course much of this material finds its way, sooner or later, to the soil; for even that which is washed into the sea may be reclaimed in sea-weed used as manure, or in fish that is used for food. But as a broad proposition, it may be assumed that practically the food of our population returns almost nothing to the soil.

The relief that the Earth-Closet offers in an agricultural point of view is not to be measured by the simple fact that it furnishes nutriment to the crop to which the manure is applied; for still greater importance attaches to the permanent benefit to the soil, resulting from any system, by which all that has been contributed to plants is surely returned. Instead of removing mineral plant-food with every crop, and sending it to the four corners of the earth, these mineral matters are returned in a form suitable for immediate use. The crop is fed, not by new contributions from the soil, but by the very material which has fed previous crops. The same elements may be used over and over again *ad infinitum.** At the same time, the action of the weather upon the soil, the

* Of course, it may or may not be the identical elements it has previously yielded which are returned to a given field, and it is not material to the argument whether it be these or their equivalent.

action of the feeding-roots of plants on the surfaces of its particles, and the power of organic matters (both the added manure and the decaying roots of previous crops) to develop latent fertilizing elements of the earth, all tend to add, year by year, to the active fertility of the land. Therefore, when the Earth System of sewage shall have been universally adopted, our fields, instead of growing poorer and poorer, as is generally the case at present, will grow constantly richer and richer; crops will grow more and more abundant; the uncertainties of cultivation will be constantly lessened; and, as the wastes of our increasing population will give an increased quantity of manure, the food of the people will constantly become more abundant and better in quality.

I once asked Mr. Horace Greeley what he thought of the Earth-Closet. His characteristic reply was, "I think that America will be "worth 25 per cent. more a hundred years hence than it would have "been without it."

All who realize the vital importance of the manure question as bearing upon the permanent prosperity of any country, will recognize the fact that, while it is impossible to measure the promise of the Earth-Closet in dollars and cents, the possibilities of its effect are almost unlimited. If we were even to admit that the domestic wastes of a population of 40,000,000 of people are worth, as manure, $400,000,000 per annum, even this would give an inadequate idea of the effect of returning to the soil not one year, but every year for evermore, everything that the soil has contributed to vegetation.

Sewage and Cess-pool Diseases.

THERE are certain grave diseases which carry off annually many thousands of our population, the causation of which has been traced with fearful clearness to what may be called, in general terms, *sewage contamination*—that is to say, they originate, directly or indirectly, in the influence of human excrement kept in undue proximity to human habitations; undergoing putrid fermentation under circumstances which allow its gases to penetrate dwelling-houses, or finding its way into wells, springs, and rivers, from which drinking-water is taken. The most notable diseases of this class are typhoid fever, gastric fever, cholera, epidemic diarrhœa, and dysentery.

Concerning typhoid fever, the Committee appointed to investigate the epidemic that broke out in the Maplewood Young Ladies' Institute, Pittsfield, Mass., in 1864, say, in their report:

"It would be impossible to bring this report within reasonable "limits, were we to discuss fully the various questions connected with "the origin and propagation of typhoid fever. Although various theo-"retical views are held as to whether the poison producing the disease "is generated in the bodies of the sick, and communicated from them "to the well, or whether it is generated in sources exterior to the bodies "of fever patients, yet all authorities maintain that a peculiar poison is "concerned in its production.

"Those who hold to the doctrine of contagion admit that, to give "such contagion efficacy in the production of wide-spread results, filth "or decaying organic matter is essential; while those who sustain the "theory of non-contagion—the production of the poison from sources "without the bodies of the sick—contend that it has its entire origin in "such filth, in decomposing matter, especially in fermenting sewage "and decaying human excreta.

"The injurious influence of decomposing azotized matter, in either "predisposing to or exciting severe disease, and particularly typhoid "fever, is universally admitted among high medical authorities."

This epidemic at Maplewood was one of the most fatal ever recorded.

"The very large proportion of so great a number of persons being "ill and having typhoid fever within so short a period points unequi- "vocally to something peculiar in their condition; to their exposure to "noxious influences of some kind, either in their locality, their diet, "or their habits. This will be more strikingly seen when the sani- "tary condition of these persons is compared with that of the com- "munity at large by which they were surrounded. Of the 74 resi- "dent pupils heard from, 66 are reported as having had illness of some "kind, at the close of the school or soon after. This is a proportion "of $\frac{33}{37}$, or nearly 90 per cent. Of these same 74, 51 had typhoid "fever, or a proportion of nearly 69 per cent. If all the people in "the town, say 8,000, had been affected in an equal proportion, more "than 7,000 would have been ill during these few weeks, and about "5,500 of them would have had typhoid fever; and of these, over "1,375 would have died. If it would be a more just comparison to take "the whole family at Maplewood into the account, estimating the "number at 112, 56 had typhoid fever, or 50 per cent.; and of these "56, 16 died, or over 28·5 per cent. These proportions, applied to "the whole population of 8,000, would give 4,000 of typhoid fever in "the same time; and of these, 1,140 would have died. According to "the testimony of the practising physicians of Pittsfield, the number of "cases of real typhoid fever, during this period, aside from those affected "by the influences at Maplewood, was small, some physicians not having "had any, others having had two or three."

From the authorities and instances cited by the Committee, I extract the following:

"Dr. E. D. Mapother, Professor of Hygiene, and Medical Officer of "Health of the city of Dublin, says: 'Typhoid fever is about the most "preventable of diseases, yet of this affection 140,000 cases occur, and "at least 20,000 young persons, including many of the flower of the "people, die every year in England.' He attributes it to foul emana- "tions, and says there is much greater risk of the disease being com- "municated from the decomposition of materials and the production of "poison in faulty sewers, than from the atmosphere about patients; "and urges the use of disinfectants, and improvements in the condition "of sewers and privies, as the preventives of this disease 'born of "putrescence.'

"One of the latest and perhaps the highest authority on this sub- "ject—Dr. Charles Murchison, of the London Fever Hospital, has ap- "plied the term 'pythogenic' (literally, 'born of putridity') to ty- "phoid fever; and, so strong is the conviction as to the particular "form of decaying matter most frequently producing it, that the name "of 'night-soil fever' has been given to it.

"In August, 1829, of 22 boys in a school at Clapham, England, 20 "were seized, within three hours, with fever, vomiting, purging, and "excessive prostration. One other boy had been seized with similar "symptoms two days before, and died comatose in 23 hours; another "boy died in 55 hours, and the rest recovered. A careful investigation "could detect no other cause than the opening and cleaning out of a "drain which had been choked up many years, and which, when open- "ed, emitted an offensive odor. This drain was at the back of the house "where the boys were, and its opening was watched by them. Its con- "tents were spread upon their play-ground. The symptoms and *post- "mortem* appearances were those of typhoid fever.

"In 1838, a circumscribed typhoid fever broke out in Birmingham, "England. About 50 cases occurred in the immediate neighborhood "of a small stream, which was nothing more than an open sewer. The "preceding season had been very hot, so that the stream was nearly "dried up, and in some places almost stagnant. It disengaged extremely "fœtid odors, especially during the night, which were complained of by "the inhabitants.

"In the same year, typhoid fever prevailed in the commune of "Prades, in the department of Ariège, France. Of 750 inhabitants, "310 were attacked, and 95 died. The cause was traced to a stagnant "pool, which was the receptacle of dead animals and of all the sewage "of the district. The outbreak was preceded by damp, warm weather. "Three times the pestilence returned, and always when the wind was "blowing over the infected water.

"In the autumn of 1857, enteric fever broke out in Fleet Lane, "London, while a sewer was being constructed. The sewer was open "from June 29 to October 30, and, during all this time, the inhabitants "complained of the offensive smell. Soon after the sewer was opened, "diarrhœa began to appear, and enteric fever followed. Of 140

" families in the lane, hardly one escaped. Those who investigated the " subject attributed the fever to sewer-miasms. It appeared soon after " the sewer was opened; it disappeared when the sewer was closed; " and, during the whole of the time, it was confined to the lane and its " immediate neighborhood.

" In the fall of 1858, an epidemic of typhoid fever prevailed at " Windsor, England. As occurring in the immediate neighborhood of " one of the royal residences, Windsor Castle, it was made a subject of " special enquiry by the medical officer of the Privy Council. Within " four months 440 persons—about one-twentieth of the whole popula- " tion—were attacked, and 39 died.

" The disease seized poor and rich alike, and the cause seemed " clearly to be traced to the escape of sewer-gases, through defects in " the drain, into the residences of the people attacked. There was a " separate sewer for the castle, which was kept in good condition, and " no case of fever occurred there. Places only a street apart, but sup- " plied respectively from the defective town-drain and the perfect " castle-drain, in the one case suffered severely, and in the other escap- " ed entirely.

" Foreign cases of this kind which have found places in the books " and journals, showing the influence of foul emanations in causing " typhoid fever, might be multiplied; but these, abstracted and con- " densed, as already intimated, from Dr. Murchison's recent and al- " most exhaustive treatise on the 'Continued Fevers of Great Britain,' " will suffice.

" Unfortunately, we have too many experiences in our own coun- " try, confirmatory of the conclusions to which the foregoing facts so " strongly tend. The National Hotel disease, which occurred at Wash- " ington, at the time of Mr. Buchanan's inauguration as President, in " 1857, is fresh in the memory of many. A large number of guests of " that popular hotel were seized, almost simultaneously, with a disease " in some respects peculiar, but essentially an intestinal or enteric fever. " Poison was suspected, but a rigorous investigation brought the com- " mittee appointed for the purpose, and all the medical attendants " upon cases, to the belief that *the disease was due to sewer-gases*. The " drain of the privy was found to be obstructed; and the foul emana- " tions were driven back, poisoning many who inhaled them. On " removing the obstructions, the effluvia and the cause of the disease " disappeared.

" Not only are these poisonous elements taken into the system in

" the air respired, but they are quite as effectual when taken into the " stomach, mingled with ingested water. The cases are numerous " where water, contaminated with fæcal and drainage matter, has been " the cause of typhoid fever and allied diseases. The following are " some of them :

" Richmond Terrace, Clifton, is a crescent composed of thirty-four " houses. In 1847, the inhabitants of thirteen of these houses drew " their drinking-water from a well at the end of the crescent. The re- " maining houses were supplied with water from another source. At " the end of September, the water of the well gave evidence to the " taste and smell of being tainted with sewage. Early in October, " *typhoid fever broke out, nearly at once, in all the thirteen houses in* " *which the tainted water had been drunk, but did not make its appear-* " *ance in any of the other houses.* In almost every one of the thirteen " houses two or three persons were ill, and in some a much larger num- " ber. The houses in which the fever broke out were far apart in the " terrace, and there was little or no intercourse between their inmates, " the water from the well being the sole connecting link.

" The following is a case even more conclusive, if possible, than " the foregoing, in demonstrating the production of typhoid fever from " foul matters—from a defective drain soaking through a porous soil into " a well, and thus contaminating the drinking-water. This case occur- " red in Williamstown, Mass.; and, as the facts have never been present- " ed in the literature of the profession, a somewhat detailed statement " will be given. Besides having had oral accounts from various entire- " ly reliable sources, the committee have received full and separate " written statements from three parties: one, a very intelligent physician " who attended many of the cases; and the other two, sufferers from the " disease, one now an advanced student of medicine, and the other of " law. One of the committee has also visited the place and examined " the premises concerned.

" From the statements, it appears that, about the middle of June, " 1860, typhoid fever broke out in a boarding-house. The whole num- " ber sitting at the table was from thirty to thirty-five persons, mostly " students of Williams College. In the course of two weeks the greater " portion of these boarders were affected—twenty or more of the stu- " dents falling sick.

" Dr. S. Duncan, one of the physicians who attended the cases " and made the investigation, says, in his communication:

" 'On the 18th of June, 1860, I was called to visit, professionally, "one of the boarders, and found him suffering with the initiatory "symptoms of typhoid fever. At this time there was, to my know- "ledge, but one case of fever in town. The patient was removed from "his lodgings in the College to this boarding-house, for the sake of "greater convenience in care and treatment, and continued to use the "water from the well on the premises for at least ten days from the first "visit.

"'This patient was under treatment for about six weeks; and, "though having, at times, unfavorable symptoms, he at length recover- "ed. About the last of June the cases began to multiply rapidly "among the boarders; and, as the disease had not made its appearance "in the town, the conviction was forced upon my own mind that its origin "was local, and that a solution of the problem might be found by an "examination of the premises. The building, cooking apparatus, and, "in fact, the whole house, was minutely inspected, without discovering "any cause for the sudden development of the disease; but out of doors "was found what was thought, at the time, to be a satisfactory explana- "tion of the phenomena.

"'A drain, which received all the refuse of the house, was found to "be choked near its exit into another drain, which conveyed surface- "water from a highly cultivated field, and which also ran near the "well. The season was uncommonly wet, and the earth in the imme- "diate neighborhood of the well was so completely saturated with "organic matter that it oozed through the ground, and stood in pools "of putrescence on the surface. Nearly two-thirds of the inmates "sickened; and, though the cases differed in severity and duration, yet "all presented the unmistakable phenomena of typhoid fever. There "were no deaths. Among the boarders were a number who did not "drink the water *at dinner*, and of these it was remarked that not one "sickened. The family of one of the professors of the College, living "in an adjoining house and using water from this well, sickened like "the others; the professor, who drank no water at dinner, alone es- "caped. I am tolerably familiar with typhoid fever, and have never "had a doubt that the disease appearing at that house, and which was "associated with drinking that water, was typhoid fever. All that "drank the water unboiled had the disease; all who avoided it in this "state escaped. It appeared that the action of heat rendered the "water innocuous, either by volatilizing, coagulating, or otherwise "changing the organic matter.'

"Though several of the students, after becoming ill, went to their "homes and suffered their sickness, no case is mentioned of the disease "having spread from them to others.

"One of the other gentlemen, in his communication, says:

"'We thought the illness was from the water:

"'(1) Because of the drain so emptying that the foul water ran "directly into the well from which we drank.

"'(2) Because, of some thirty or thirty-five boarders, all at the "same table, those who drank tea and coffee exclusively three times "a day (and there were several such) escaped all symptoms; as well "as those who took ale for dinner, and tea and coffee at the morning "and the evening meal.

"'(3) It could not have arisen from impure air, study, or epidemic "influence, as none in the town were affected save parties who used "the water; and many who were sick were among the *laziest* of "students.

"'(4) Those were the subjects of the severest sickness who were "exclusively drinkers of water. One of the sick, who never used any "other drink, was confined eight weeks, and was unable to fill his ap-"pointment on commencement-day.

"'Another, who drank water moderately, and only at dinner, had "the disease in a much milder form, and was confined a very much "shorter time.'

"This gentleman, the writer of the account, was seized on the 25th "of June, and he says:

"'At, or within a day or two previous to and after, my illness, "several of the boarders were seized with similar symptoms and sent "home.'

"From these dates, it appears that the cases continued to occur "from near the time of the attack of the first until all were affected. "Some resisted the influence of the water longer than others, but all "were taken within a period of ten days. The water, when carefully "noticed, was found to taste and smell of the sewage; though, when "served upon the table with ice, these qualities were not perceived.

"Although this poison is sometimes conveyed to the system through "the medium of drinking-waters, yet in most cases it is taken through "the air. Says Dr. Murchison: 'Many instances might be cited where, "although the water supply was the same to all, only those persons "exposed to sewer-emanations have been attacked.'

"The intimate connection between typhoid fever and night-soil, "sewer-emanations, or contaminated drinking-waters is now so gene-

"rally recognized by the more enlightened members of the profession, "that, so far as they are concerned, some even of these citations might "have been omitted; but so much ignorance prevails in the community "at large on this subject that these references to facts and authorities "are deemed necessary for the purposes of this report."

The following, concerning typhoid fever, is taken from "Notes on Epidemics," by Dr. Anstie:

"Of exciting causes, two are recognized as outweighing in import- "ance all the rest. The first is the direct introduction of decomposing "organic matters (and possibly of organic germs developed from this "source) into the alimentary canal, by the agency of impure drinking- "water; and, secondly, the inhalation of the gases formed in the decom- "position of organic matters, and possibly specific germs along with "these. Of the former mode of origin it is easy to find countless ex- "amples in the medical history of our country towns. . . . The "following are the typical conditions in which typhoid fever arises from "impurities in drinking-water (we write with a well-remembered instance "in our mind). A country town, without deep drainage, disposes of "its sewage in cess-pools; and the limited space in which the houses "stand renders it inevitable that the drinking-wells should be within a "very short distance of the cess-pools. From the latter a continual ooz- "ing of decomposing organic matters takes place, and more or less of "these finds its way into the wells. For years, possibly, no particular "harm can result from this, but at length there comes a long, dry sum- "mer, which reduces the water to a low ebb, and concentrates its impu- "rities, besides favoring decomposition. In such circumstances, typhoid "fever breaks out among the persons who drink the water.

"Such is the story which scores of country towns have repeated in "their own experience. But there is another mode of origin of which "we possess examples of apparently equal accuracy. A hot, dry season "favors decomposition, as we have already said; under these circum- "stances, sewage gases ascend through the imperfect traps of the drains "into the interior of the houses; and of this, also, an outbreak of ty- "phoid is of frequent consequence. . . . In short, all observers "arrive at the conclusion, that it would be possible, by rendering "our drinking-water absolutely pure, and by disinfecting our sewage "at the earliest moment, almost or entirely to suppress typhoid "fever."

The following extracts are taken from three different papers, read by Ed. C. C. Stanford, F.C.S.*

First paper:

" No system of sewerage is worthy our consideration which does not " give back to the soil that which in our food we have taken from it; " and I consider the mere ridding ourselves of a valuable fertilizer, " simply on account of difficulty in dealing with it, quite beneath the " enlightened spirit of our age. . . .

" And as to the sewer-gases, it appears, according to the evidence " collected by the Sewage Commission, quite impossible to get rid of " them; one of the engineers examined making this terribly suggestive " answer:

" 'I am afraid we must let out the stink in the middle of the " streets.'

" Now, stink is not the word, for sewer-gases are gases of decompo- " sition, and carry malaria, pestilence, and death with them. Dr. Fer- " gus has related one of many instances in which a number of houses at " Leith, previously healthy, have been affected *at once* with gastric (or " typhoid) fever when connected with the sewers; and showing the " constant infiltration of sewage into the soil, and thence into wells; he " has also pointed out cases of gastric fever where the long-unsuspected " cause was the drinking of the water so contaminated. . . .

" The water-closet system is also open to great objection; the best " constructed closet is seldom perfectly free from odor; the back rush of " deadly gases up the sewers, when a high tide covers them or a strong " gale blows into their outlets at low tide, is of enormous force, and will " rise through any closet, however well trapped.

" Water is a mere carrier, and no disinfectant; its cost, also, from " the great quantity required, is very considerable. . . .

" The whole system of sewerage by water-carriage is extravagant. " It carries the solid and liquid excreta down to our neighbors to rot at " their doors, and it leaves us a legacy of deadly gases to remind us " that our endeavor to cheat nature has signally failed. As applied to " even ridding ourselves of the nuisance, it is the finest effort of the " 'circumlocution office,' and the best illustration of 'how not to do it' " in our generation.

" Engineers have employed an elephant to do the work of a

* The first before the Glasgow Sewage Association, March 30, 1868; the second before the Chemical Section of the Glasgow Philosophical Society, April 19, 1869; the third before the British Association, 1869.

" mouse, and the burly brute has trodden down and laid waste the " country."

Mr. Stanford takes up the subject of Earth Sewage, and shows its great superiority to the water system, but finds objection to it in the large quantity of earth required, suggesting, as a better material, charred sea-weed. He seems not to have been informed as to the great saving of earth that is effected by repeated using.

Professor Joy estimates that *one cubic foot* of earth *per annum* is sufficient for the use of each individual, if it is systematically redried and used eight times over, which is entirely practicable, and which brings the system of Earth Sewage, with all its advantages in the matter of health, comfort, and economy, within the reach of the largest towns.

Second paper:

" . . . In the paper referred to, I endeavored to show that, " whatever may be the best, *the present water-closet system, with all its* " *boasted advantages, is the worst that can be generally adopted;* briefly, " because it is a most extravagant method of converting a mole-hill into " a mountain. It merely removes the bulk of our excreta from our " cities to choke our rivers with foul deposit and rot at our neighbors' " doors. It increases the death-rate as well as all other rates, and intro- " duces into our houses a most deadly enemy in the shape of sewer " gases.

" . . . The water-closet, with many apparent advantages, " and with all our prejudices in its favor, carries an attendant train of " evils which I am fully persuaded will ultimately doom it to obli- " vion. . . .

" . . . During the past year, Moule's Dry Closet has been " largely introduced; all who have used it speak in the highest terms of " its efficiency, and there are already strong indications of its becoming " the system of the future.

" . . . Our authorities want, of course, some grand scheme; " but they forget that the question is one of minute details. We are " assailed by a large army of small nuisances—one, at least, to every " house, and we must attack them one at a time. Attacked in their " united strength, they will assuredly overcome us. Ought we not rather " to strike at the root of the evil? Ought we not to stop the mischief "at its numerous sources, and before these can combine into a mighty "force which carries everything before it?

"Let the subject be calmly and carefully discussed; let us not be "carried away by great schemes and useless expenditure; let us not "leave to posterity heavy taxes, with barren wastes and desolate cities; "but let us rather pay our own way, and leave our country fertile and "our towns pure, and I shall never regret that, however imperfectly "this subject has been brought before you, my earnest wish has been to "strike 'one more blow for life.'"

Third paper:

"In these papers, I have endeavored to show that the water-closet "system of disposing of human excreta can never be regarded as the "perfect system of the future. I have strongly urged the general adop-"tion of the Dry Closet as avoiding all the great evils which are appa-"rently inseparable from the use of water as a vehicle; and pointed out "the use of charcoal, by which its application to towns and cities is "simple and easy. . . .

"Amongst other objections to the use of water as a carrier, I have "specified:

"1. The enormous cost of the works required, in proportion to the "small amount of noxious material to be removed.

"2. The large annual outlay required to keep the closets in order. "Experience in large cities has shown that, on this account, these closets "are quite unsuitable for the dwellings of the poor.

"3. The enormous amount of water employed (estimated at 365 "times the weight of the excreta), whereas in many towns there is much "difficulty in obtaining it.

"4. That it results in a subterranean flood of filthy water, which "must flow somewhere; and wherever it flows it pollutes the region, "thus disseminating and distributing the evil.

"5. This material, worth about 30*s.* per ton. has its value reduced "by dilution to 1*d.* per ton, which it is impossible, by any known chemi-"cal method, to extract with profit.

"6. The large generation of noxious gases in the sewers, which "constantly escape into our streets and houses.

"In reference to the latter, Dr. Gairdner speaks strongly of almost "all sewers as 'diffusing poisons upwards and downwards,' and too "often 'carrying backwards into the very heart of the dwelling the "reflux gases, the produce of the decomposition of the impurities of a "whole neighborhood.'

"Dr. Fergus characterizes the sewers as 'a gigantic laboratory under "our dwellings,' from which noxious gases escape by gully-holes into "our streets, and pipes into our houses.

"He has furnished me with a number of extracts from eminent "medical authorities, which conclusively show the highly dangerous "character of the miasma occasioned by the infiltration of sewage-"water and the evolution of sewer-gas.

"Of these I shall only make two quotations, which should be suffi-"cient to convince any one of the important bearing of this question on "the national health.

"EXTRACT I.—*Mr. Simm's Second Report* (1860) *of Dr. Greenhow's* "*Investigations in several towns in England*, pp. 59 and 60:

"'*Diarrhœal diseases* are increasing in this country; they vary in dif-"ferent districts from 4 to 663 per 100,000 persons. If the diarrhœal "death-rate of England generally were only ten times the minimum "death-rate, there would be an annual saving in England of nearly "20,000 lives.

"'In the districts which suffer the high diarrhœal death-rates, the "population either breathes or drinks a larger amount of putrefying "animal refuse.'

"Page 61: 'If the diarrhœal death-rate of England is reduced to "that which prevails among the healthier parts of the population, ty-"phoid fever (now probably the cause of at least 15,000 annual deaths) "will probably be reduced in more than equal measure; and in propor-"tion as infantile diarrhœa is reduced, the convulsive disorders and "respiratory inflammations of infancy (which now cause fully 60,000 "annual deaths) will also show a large if not equal reduction of death-"rates.'

"Page 64: 'The excess of mortality has in all cases been coinci-"dent with one or other of two local circumstances: (*a*) *The tainting of* "*the atmosphere with the products of organic decomposition, especially of hu-*"*man excrement;* or (*b*) *The habitual drinking of impure water.*'

"EXTRACT II.—From *Mr. Simon's Ninth Report to the Privy* "*Council*, pp. 32–34:

"'*Cholera* derives all its epidemic destructiveness from filth, and "especially from excremental uncleanliness.

"'It cannot be too distinctly understood that the person who con-"tracts cholera in this country is, *ipso facto*, demonstrated, with almost "absolute certainty, to have been exposed to excremental pollution; "that what gave him cholera was, mediately or immediately, cholera "contagion discharged from another's bowels; that, in short, this diffu- "sion of cholera among us depends entirely on the numberless filthy "facilities which are let exist, and especially in our larger towns, for the "fouling of earth and air and water, and thus, secondarily, for the infec- "tion of man with whatever contagion may be contained in the miscel- "laneous outflowings of the population. Excrement-sodden earth, ex- "crement-reeking air, excrement-tainted water, these are for us the "causes of cholera. Cholera ravaging here at long intervals is not "nature's only retribution for our neglect of such matters as are in "question. *Typhoid fever and much endemic diarrhœa are, as I have* "*often reported, incessant witnesses to the same deleterious influences. Ty-* "*phoid fever, which annually kills from* 15,000 *to* 20,000 *of our popula-* "*tion; and diarrhœa, which kills many thousands besides.*'

"None of the disadvantages enumerated attend the use of the Dry "Closet; still less can any of these gigantic malaria evils result from its "general adoption. *It meets every sanitary requirement*, which, after "all, is the main consideration. Moreover, its machinery is simple and "inexpensive. It effects at once a great saving of water; and it enables "us to secure the whole of the value of the excreta. I have pointed out "the only objections which can be urged against its application in large "cities to be, when dry earth is used, the large amount required (three "and a half times the weight of the excreta), the difficulty of obtaining "such a supply, and the large cartage necessary. . . .

"I admit that considerations of health must always precede those "of wealth in this respect, and no system need be spoken of against "which there is a whisper of suspicion on this point.

"*Nothing can be said against the Dry Closet in this respect.* It has "already become a recognized institution. It presents the best means "at present known of confining a nuisance within its proper limits, "instead of distributing it amongst our neighbors, and therefore merits "our patient consideration. There can be no doubt that for country- "houses the Earth-Closet is free from objection."

It is accepted as a fact that cholera is propagated mainly, if not entirely, by either the exhalation into the air of the resultant gases of the decomposition of the fæces of cholera patients, or by the leaking into wells of the soluble parts of such fæces.

As a consequence, *poisoned air* and *poisoned drinking-water* are the recognized agents in the causation of the disease; and the practice, common in all country towns, of either discharging water-closets into leaking or overflowing cess-pools, or of using the common privy-vault, leads directly to the propagation of cholera as an epidemic disease.

Dr. Anstie, in his " Notes on Epidemics," says (p. 53): " The year " 1854 was made memorable in the annals of medical science by the re- " markable outbreak of cholera in the parish of St. James, Westminster. " The disease had already announced its presence by the occurrence of " a few cases during the latter months of 1853; but the number of " attacks declined, in the two first quarters of 1854, to a very low ebb; " at the end of June, however, they began to increase, till, in the last " week of September, the cholera mortality reached 2,050. In the " parish of St. James, the first fatal case for 1854 happened at the end " of July; but there was only a dropping fire, as it were, which kept " within quite moderate limits up to the last days of August, when sud- " denly the disease made an enormous explosion in the district. In the " most crowded part of this densely crowded parish there occurred, on " the 31st of August, no less than *thirty-one* fatal cases, all within an ex- " tremely narrow area: on the following day there were 131 fatal cases " in the same area; on the 2d September, 125; on the 3d, 58; on the " 4th, 52; on the 5th, 26; on the 6th, 28; on the 7th, 22; on the 8th, " 14 fatal attacks, all in the same space, which might be marked off by " a circle . . . whose radius would be of the length of 210 yards. . . .

" Fixing his attention on the local peculiarities of the district, Dr. " Snow quickly perceived that one remarkable circumstance was com- " mon to the history of the large majority of attacks of the disease, " namely, that the sufferers had been in the habit of drinking the water of " a well in Broad Street, which had a great reputation for sweetness and " freshness. Analysis of this water soon showed that it was highly " charged with organic impurities; and, on the 8th of September, the " vestry, on the urgent persuasion of Dr. Snow, removed the handle of " the pump, and so prevented the further use of the well. On subse- " quent examination, it was discovered that the sewage from a neigh- " boring house-drain had leaked into the well, and that the discharge of " a patient residing in the house in question, and suffering from severe " diarrhœa, if not from actual cholera, must have mingled with the sew- " age immediately before the date of the great epidemic outbreak."

Anstie further says (p. 62): " It is now well established that this " affection (epidemic diarrhœa) is caused by the effluvia from the de-

" composition of organic matter, or by the admixture of such impurities " with drinking-water." P. 65: "The diseases of which we have been " treating certainly owe their propagation chiefly to sewer-gases in the " air, and sewage matters mixed with food or drink."

" Pettenkofer's observations appear to prove decidedly that the " drinking-water had no inconsiderable share in the propagation of cho- " lera in the epidemic at Munich. But they further demonstrate very " clearly that the situation of houses on a porous soil of any kind en- " sured a greatly increased rapidity and energy of diffusion of the " disease; while rocky foundations afforded a very remarkable protec- " tion from the same. Pettenkofer was convinced by ample evidence " that the penetration of the soil by the discharges of cholera patients " was the first essential link in the chain of propagation, and the coinci- " dence of this part of his theory with Snow's affords a strong support to " it. The further stage, however, was considered by the Bavarian pro- " fessor to consist not in the defilement of the drinking-water, but in the " formation of a miasmatic vapor of the decomposing matter, which " vapor conveyed the poison by inhalation to the lungs of the in- " habitants of the houses.

" There appears to us no reason for rejecting either theory. . . .

" Epidemic diarrhœa is the constant product in this country of " autumnal seasons, which succeed to a long continuance of hot, dry " summer weather. It is now well established that this affection is " caused by the effluvia from decomposing organic matter, or by the ad- " mixture of such impurities with drinking-water."

After ascribing a similar cause to the propagation of dysentery, Dr. Anstie cites the following instance, which should attract the attention of the authorities of country towns in which night-soil is spread on the surface of the ground as a manure, without being previously disinfected:

" The first is one that occurred last year at a lunatic asylum: this " establishment was surrounded by fields, the cultivation of which form- " ed an interesting and very valuable occupation for many of the unfor- " tunate inmates of the asylum. It was determined to test upon these " fields the value of liquid sewage as a fertilizing manure, and, accord- " ingly, large quantities of the sewage matters supplied by the house " were applied to this economic purpose. Unfortunately, it happened " that a large part of the ground so treated lay very near to the windows "of the asylum, and the wind carried the gases from the decomposing "organic matters into the house; the result was an outbreak of very "severe and fatal dysenteric diarrhœa. It was immediately pointed "out by various medical men that all this mischief might have been "avoided by disinfecting the sewage matters before discharging them "on the land; meantime, the harm had been done."

In the *Lancet*, of March 6, 1869, Professor Rolleston set forth some objections to the Earth-Closet system, in the course of which he said:

"'If I am told that the earth-closet is inoffensive and that the privy "is fœtid, I answer that a rattlesnake is none the less dangerous because "its rattle is removed; and that, for anything shown or known to the "contrary, odor is to infection, deodorization to disinfection, what the "noise of the serpent is to its bite.' He adds the results of five scienti- "fic experiments, and, anticipating apparently the conclusions which "even professional readers would draw from them, says, 'It will be "asked, Do not these experiments show that ashes and earth are, each of "them in their respective order, superior to water for use in closets?' "and goes on to give various reasons why he *thinks* otherwise."

The following reply appears in the *Lancet*, from the Rev. Henry Moule, of Fordington Vicarage:

"With all respect for so high an authority as Dr. Rolleston, I beg "permission to offer to your readers the following remarks on his article "in this week's *Lancet*, on the 'Earth-Closet System.' That letter, "grounded on an inadequate conception of the system, grievously mis- "represents it; for it either denies or ignores its merits, and an efficacy, "which the experience of several years (and that for some time past ex- "tending into every variety of climate) proves it to possess. And it "ascribes to it evils from which that same experience renders it in the "highest degree probable that it is entirely free. The main evil of the "privy-vault, of the cess-pool, and of the common sewer is found in the "accumulation of excreta; and that under circumstances which almost "immediately and continuously necessitate fermentation and the gene- "ration of the most deleterious gases. This can be dealt with only in "the mass; and universal experience proves the almost, if not entire, "impossibility under such circumstances of dealing with it effectually. "Whereas, in the most direct contradistinction to this, the Dry Earth "system deals with excreta *at once* and *in detail*, and thus cuts off the evil "at its source. Three half-pints of dry earth, powdered or finely sifted, "thrown immediately on a single evacuation, will prevent the escape "into the room or closet of all offensive smell or deleterious gas. All "vapor or gas that the excreta exhale is taken into the earth covering "it; and the finer the earth the more complete the interpenetration of "the two substances. More than this, we by this means prevent fer-"mentation; and with this is prevented any approach to emission of "sulphuretted hydrogen. And so complete in both cases is this result, "that the deposit with repeated additions may remain in the pail, or iron "tank, or dry brick vault, into which it falls, in the same innoxious state "for weeks or months. Or it may be immediately removed from the "chamber without offensiveness or injury, and deposited in a shed for "drying. And when sufficiently dry it may in that state be safely trans-"ported to any distance, and handed over to the gardener or farmer— "and that either in the loamy valley or the rocky soil of the mountain— "as a valuable manure. And after countless experiments and observa-"tions during ten years, I feel quite confident that throughout the several "stages of this process 'the rattlesnake' will injure no one. For he has "not only lost his 'rattle' by deodorization, but, by absorption, by the "entire absence of fermentation, and by the most minute mechanical and "chemical disintegration, he has either been strangled in his birth or torn "into ten thousand atoms. Now, what does Dr. Rolleston in his letter "set against all this? First, he gives Von Pettenkofer's opinion, which, "even if resting on a better foundation, is, strange to say, quite irrelevant "to the subject against which it is adduced. Von Pettenkofer says: "'I cannot see my way towards recommending the disinfection of "privies with earth and peat.' But to disinfect privies and cess-pools is "no part of the Dry Earth system. Its great object is not to disinfect "but to supersede those abominations, and the equal abomination of the "sewer. But if the opinion be thus irrelevant, so must be that which "Dr. Rolleston grounds on it, respecting the localization and diffusion of "typhoid fever. And equally irrelevant are his remarks on the compa-"rative dangers of the contaminated well and the bespattered privy. "Now even if the question were doubtful as to these, the prevention of "the contamination of wells would be a desirable object. And this the "Dry Earth system effects. At the same time it obviates the offensive-"ness of the 'bespattered privies.' I scarcely need remark on Baron "Liebig's conjectural system of the removal of sewage by water as placed "in competition with the Dry Earth system now in so many hundred "places successfully established. And against Dr. Rolleston's five ex-

"periments in his laboratory several times repeated, whatever may be "their scientific value, I am content to set the five years' experience of "the Dry Earth system throughout the whole of British India. Surely, "if Dr. Rolleston's apprehensions be just, we ought ere this to have "heard of outbreaks of cholera or fever in jails with 700 and even 1,500 "inmates, in which this system during those five years has been in full "operation. I have heard of none. I cannot ask for space to remark "on the difficulties which Dr. Rolleston expresses on the working of a "system, with which either in its fulness or its details he seems to be so "imperfectly acquainted. I would, in conclusion, express my surprise "that the only extract given from Dr. Mouat's 'Report on the Jails of the "Lower Provinces of India,' should be that which is in fact a caution "against a hasty deposition beneath the soil of the removed excreta and "earth. And I would ask Dr. Rolleston and your readers to place by "the side of that extract, and of all that he has written, the following "passage, written by the same eminent officer in that very same report: "'It is impossible, in my humble opinion, to overestimate the result of "the Rev. Mr. Moule's labors in this important branch of hygiene—the "Dry Earth system. It is without exception the greatest public benefit "conferred by a private individual in a matter so essential to public "health, that I am acquainted with.'"

I have, at the risk of being tiresome, gone more fully into the question of infection, and the propagation of disease, than may seem to have been necessary in advocating the reform under consideration. But I believe that there is no statement in all of the foregoing extracts that it is not of vital consequence to every intelligent person to consider.

The preservation of health and the arresting of infectious diseases are the first duty of us all, whether regard is had to the sanitary arrangements of our own houses or of the communities of which we form a part. We have no right either to so keep our household wastes as to endanger the health of our families, or to deposit them, whether by sewer transportation or otherwise, where they will endanger the health of other people. If, therefore, the reader has passed over any part of these extracts from medical authorities, I beg that he will apply himself again to the task, and attain a full realization of the evils from which the Earth-Closet System, and it alone, has power to give relief.

THE DRY-EARTH SYSTEM

FOR

CITIES AND TOWNS.

WHEN my attention was first called to the subject of the Earth-Closet, and during my earlier experience with it, I regarded it only as a most feasible and promising reform for introduction into country houses and country towns, as a substitute for water-closets (which can hardly be said to be available under such circumstances), and of the disgraceful common privy. The extension of the system to large cities, or under any circumstances where public water supply and sewerage are provided, seemed impracticable even if desirable; and it is only as I have gained more knowledge of the subject that I have come to believe that the water-closet, instead of being a blessing, is only a " curse in " disguise;" that every consideration of economy and health demands its abandonment; and that there is no reason why, even in the most densely peopled cities, the use of the Earth-Closet may not become universal.

It is so much cheaper, and so much less liable to get out of order and to need expensive repairs, that its use would relieve landlords and tenants of an onerous tax, while its greater efficiency, and its far greater ability to withstand abuse without becoming dangerously offensive, are such that, if the single difficulty of earth supply and removal were obviated, its use would extend almost as fast as the conviction of its advantages.

It will be found, by computation, that this difficulty is much less serious than at first would be supposed. For instance, let us assume that this system is in universal use in the city of New York, with a population of 800,000. Under these circumstances, there will probably be 1,200,000 uses of the closet per day. This would require, according to Professor Joy's estimate, 50,000 cubic feet of earth, or about 2,000 one-horse cart-loads. With proper arrangements in convenient situations for redrying and sifting the earth, so that each lot should be used five times, 400 loads of fresh earth would have to be brought into the city for every day's use; and, if the waste and evaporation counterbalanced the solid dry matter of the fæces, an equal amount for each day would have to be removed.

By this computation, if the annual voidings of each person are valued at $5, each load taken out after five uses would be worth $27. This would allow $2 for the first cost of the earth, and $5 for each handling.

Basing the calculation upon Mr. Moule's estimate of 1½ lbs. for each use, the daily requirement would be 900 tons; or, if used five times over, 180 tons; or, eight times over, 112 tons. By these calculations, the manure being worth $5 per individual, the manure, after five uses, would be worth $60 per ton, and, after eight uses, $97 per ton, allowing fully $12 per ton for each handling.

There can be no doubt whatever that earth which has been used five times in the Closet will find a ready sale at $50 per ton (for it is usual in England to estimate its value after seven uses as equal to that of Peruvian guano, which sells at about $80 in New York). This will allow $2 per ton for the original cost of the earth, and $6 for each handling, which would be fully three times its actual cost, including the rent of proper storage-room.

The above calculations will show that, even in a compactly built large city like New York, the complete introduction of the Dry Earth System would be not only feasible, but enormously profitable, even if it had to depend entirely on earth brought from a distance; but New York need not depend on this; it is quite possible that no earth at all need be brought in. The testimony of Professor Jackson and others is very clear as to the entire efficiency of coal-ashes; and my own experiments with these have shown that the only objection to their use is to be found in the dust that accompanies their disturbance. This would hardly be a practicable objection under any ordinary circumstances. The dust that would arise in filling the hopper of a Commode, would not be greater than in cleaning a parlor grate. If this material should be found by extended experiment to answer all of the requirements, the problem for cities would be solved. The unconsumed fuel in ashes would well pay for their sifting, and the quantity made by the fires of any household would be ample for the use of its closets. Should this source of absorbent material prove to be sufficient, the removal of the fæces of the city would not add materially to the present cost of removing the ashes, while the manurial value that these would acquire would be an important source of revenue.

I offer it as a suggestion merely that the quality of the manure and the satisfactory working of the closets might be increased if the dirt of the streets were mixed with the ashes, and the whole material dried and sifted preparatory to use. If this should prove feasible, it would greatly simplify the street-cleaning problem, and return to the soil not only the excrement of the population, but that of the immense number of horses as well.

Of course, I am not so Quixotic as to suppose that the Earth-Closet will, for a very long time, if ever, be generally adopted in the more densely peopled parts of the city; but the whole area above the lower end of the Central Park is exactly suited for its introduction. The whole Harlem flat is so low and level that it will be almost impossible to lay the sewers so high as not to be entered by salt-water at high tide, and, in any event, it will hardly be practicable to give them sufficient fall to remove with certainty anything but the pure water of surface drainage. The offensiveness of the ordinary gaseous emanations from sewers is greatly enhanced by an admixture of salt-water; and if the sewer system now in use shall be the only reliance in One Hundred and Seventh Street, for instance, when it is closely built up from Fifth Avenue to the River, it will probably be the most disagreeable and most unhealthy street in the civilized world.

Nearly all of the northern part of the Island that is not included in the Harlem flat has the rock so near to the surface that the opening of trenches for large sewers must be a work of enormous expense, and the rock itself is so seamed with fissures that leakage from the sewers would in many cases find its way beneath the houses.

If the Dry Earth system of sewage is possible in New York, the arguments in its favor would be stronger, and the objections to its use fewer, in almost every other city in the country. Philadelphia, Chicago, St. Louis, Memphis, New Orleans, Savannah, Charleston, and Washington can, it seems to me, be perfectly cleansed of their human wastes in no other way. Philadelphia is much better than the others, but even there the introduction of the system would be as beneficent as the carrying out of its details would be easy. Chicago now voids its filth into a sluggish river, lying in the heart of the city, which in summer is almost absolutely without current, and its offensiveness is well-nigh past endurance, while its fatal influence as a source of disease can hardly be overestimated. St. Louis can be sewered only at enormous expense, and it is surrounded with worn-out tobacco and hemp lands, to which the earth manure would be a godsend. Three-fourths of the future great city of Memphis must empty its sewers into the Gayoso Bayou, where, during the summer months, unless fresh water is pumped into it from the Mississippi, it will produce a condition even worse, if possible, than Chicago River already causes. In New Orleans, sewage is impossible. Both graves and privy-vaults are built on the top of the moist soil. Water-closets are unknown, and the cleansing of the vaults is an expensive and annoying necessity. Of the topography of Savannah I have no personal knowledge, but I am informed that it is not materially different from that of Charleston, whose sewers are a mockery, and impress a stranger rather as receptacles for offensive black mud (to be taken out through man-holes into the street) than as a means for carrying away the wastes of the town.

The condition of affairs in Washington is described to me by a Justice of one of the United States Courts as being, beyond expression, bad. The soil being a heavy clay filled with moisture, privy-vaults must be built above the surface of the ground, or, in every heavy rain, their fœtid contents will overflow. Water-closets are very unsatisfactory, even where the supply of water is provided for, because, the sewers of the avenues belonging to the United States, and those of the streets to the city authorities, there is always a difficulty about making connections; and the town generally is not creditable, in respect to its sanitary arrangements, to the "highly civilized" people whose capital it is.

As we descend the scale and come to towns of smaller size, the condition of affairs grows worse rather than better. As an example, let us take this very town of Newport, which is not only a fashionable watering-place, but a tidy, quiet, well-built, well-to-do town, of from 12,000 to 15,000 inhabitants. Setting aside its $100,000 "cottages," the town itself is remarkably well built. It gives far more evidence of comfortable and decent living, in proportion to the number of its habitations, than any other town with which I am acquainted. So far as one can judge from its outward appearance, it hardly ranks second to any other town in New England in cleanliness and good order. But in the matter of its closet accommodations, among both rich and poor, it is simply vile. Those houses that are provided with water-closets have also most offensive and dangerous cess-pools in close proximity to them. Common old-fashioned vaults are almost universal. They are excavated in a heavy, wet, undrained clay soil, and are filled nearly to overflowing during the greater part of the year with a liquid mass of filth, that is worse than the contents of even the most offensive dry vault, and more pernicious, I believe, in its influence on health.

It is reported, I know not with what accuracy, that in 1863, in consequence of the overflowing or springing a leak of the cess-pool of one of the large hotels, a most fatal epidemic was spread through all that part of the town of which the drinking-water wells lies within reach of the same water-bearing strata.

The almost incessant winds prevailing here probably prevent the spread of the influence of these vaults and cess-pools by atmospheric contamination. But the impervious soil is stratified with porous veins of sand and gravel, through which the interchange of contents between wells and privy-vaults is in many cases facilitated.

The farmers of Rhode Island, having a keen appreciation of the value of manure, haul the entire contents of these vaults (in a state of very thin dilution), and spread them on their fields, and during the winter season, when the work is going on, these abominations are constantly met moving through the streets in broad daylight, creating an offence that realizes one's worst ideas of Chinese nastiness. The effect on the senses of a ride among the fields to which this manure is applied as a broadcast top-dressing may be imagined.

Newport is by no means exceptional in these respects. I have referred to it more particularly only because the details of its condition have come under my own observation. Probably the majority of towns in America of the same size are in at least as ill regulated a condition; but I am glad to believe that, whatever may be done in the large cities, these smaller towns (which are now dreaming of aqueducts, reservoirs, and sewers) will, within a few years, be completely provided for by means of the Earth Sewage, and will become in reality, what they now appear to be, worthy abodes of intelligent and civilized people.

THE DETAILS OF EARTH SEWAGE.

BEFORE the Earth System can be adopted into general use, the slight care and attention that its success requires must be accepted as an addition to the details of domestic and municipal economy.

The water system, with its enormous bills of expense for reservoirs, aqueducts, service-pipes, plumbing work, and sewers, requires constant supervision and care. Whether in private establishments in the country or in large cities, the details of its management require an amount of supervision and of costly labor which, could they have been set forth before the system was anywhere introduced, would have seemed an insuperable objection to its adoption. Now, they are taken as a matter of course, and water-rates and sewer commissioners' taxes are accepted as a necessity of civilized life, and are paid without demur.

The Earth System promises to do away with the necessity for most of these charges, and to produce a money result which will more than repay the others.

At the same time, the perfect carrying out of the Earth System of sewage will require a certain amount of care and some expense, which it will be better to consider at the outset. It is not worth while to make a comparison between the requirements of the two rivals, because the more vital considerations, according to which the verdict is to be given, are so weighty that the question of relative cost is comparatively insignificant. If, as I believe is proven, the Earth System is more conducive than the water system to health and economy, it will inevitably, sooner or later, become universal in its application.

There are two extreme cases to be considered, and the various conditions that fill the gap between them will necessarily resemble one or the other according to their magnitude. In all cases, the *principles* are identical.

1. The earth for use in closets must be dry; not necessarily dried by artificial heat, but made as dry as it can be by exposure to the air and by the exclusion of rain.

2. It must contain enough alumina (clay), or organic matter, or oxide of iron to give it sufficient absorbing power.

3. It must be sifted of its stones and coarser particles.

4. The mechanical arrangement of the closet must be such that a sufficient quantity of earth will be, with certainty, deposited upon the fæces—enough to cover them, and to absorb the urine of the single evacuation. And the accumulation under the seat must be occasionally raked down or levelled off in the vault.

5. When the vault or receptacle has become too full, its contents must be removed, and before the supply is exhausted the reservoir must be refilled.

6. If the earth is to be again used, its organic matter must be destroyed by fermentation, and its moisture must be evaporated.

7. In towns, some system must be adopted (similar to that proposed for Riverside) for the supply of earth and removal of deposits—either by the public authorities or by private enterprise.

1. As Mr. Moule very tersely states the case, "An Earth-Closet "will no more work without *Dry Earth* than a water-closet will work " without water;" but the dryness here referred to is not absolute dryness, for the earth of the closet will always contain what moisture may be absorbed from the atmosphere. This, and even a little more than this, I have found to be not at all objectionable. What is required is, according to Professor Joy, that so much of the moisture of the fæces shall be immediately withdrawn from them that there shall be too little left to cause an offensive putrefaction.

The best manner for drying the earth depends very much upon the quantity required, and the means at command. Two or three cart-loads, which will be sufficient for a year's use of an ordinary family, may be taken from a ploughed field or a road-side gutter during the dry weather of summer. Dumped in an out-of-the-way corner under a wood-shed, or in any other dry place, being underlaid with boards to prevent it from absorbing the moisture of the earth, it will soon become sufficiently dry for use, and will remain so throughout the dampest and foggiest weather of the winter or spring. It might be equally well-kept in a dry and well-ventilated cellar. It may be sifted, little by little, as wanted, and it will answer tolerably well if it is merely put through the ordinary coal-sifter, though something finer would be preferable. My sieve has six meshes to the inch; perhaps four would do as well. When the earth is sifted, it may be stowed away in boxes or barrels in some easily accessible place, and there remain until wanted for use. This is sufficient for the requirements of a private house.

In preparing for the supply of a large town, it would be necessary to procure a land-right in order that deep excavations can be made The amount of earth needed will be very large, and it must, of course, be procured in the cheapest way. This will be, in nearly all cases, by making a clean sweep as deep as it is economical to work, and making an acre of land produce as much earth as possible. The high price of land in the immediate vicinity of the town may make it desirable to go to a considerable distance, in order to secure cheap land and cheap transportation combined. The earth being procured, the first drying can be most economically done near the spot from which it was taken, by simply storing it under rain-tight and well-ventilated sheds. The drier it becomes the less water is to be transported; and, to avoid the danger of wetting *in transitu*, the earth should be sifted and packed in barrels before leaving the sheds. It would, perhaps, be well to make some provision for rapid, artificial drying in the town to provide against emergency and accident.

2. There is undoubtedly a good deal of difference in the effectiveness of earths of various composition; though, with a considerable range of experiment and observation, I am inclined to think that the kinds of earth which are *not* suited for use in the Closet are much fewer than

would be generally supposed. Pure sand and gravel are worthless, but I think that any earth that contains enough clay or organic matter for the production of ordinary crops will answer the purpose. A nearly pure clay, however, is objectionable from its tendency to absorb moisture from the air. If to be used only once, an equal weight of muck or peat may be, from its greater bulk, more valuable than clay. The clay could probably be used many more times, and so would be cheaper for use in towns. Without being able to give a definite scientific reason for the opinion, I think that a clay loam, highly charged with oxides of iron (notably reddish clay loams), would be the best.

Mr. Stanford, whose articles I have quoted from the *Chemical News*, very strongly urges the use of some form of animal or sea-weed charcoal for use in towns; but it seems to me that it is not necessary to seek for anything better than a suitable earth, and that an attempt to supply all the towns in the United States with such charcoal would be defeated by the great price that so general a demand would cause.

3. The sifting of the earth is, as I have shown, a very simple matter when it is a question merely of the supply of a single household. When large quantities are required, it would be the most economical plan to adopt revolving screens, such as are used for cleaning coal at mines, the construction being similar to that of the bolting screen of a common flour-mill. Such a screen should be, probably, twenty feet long, the first half of its length being furnished with quarter-inch meshes, and the next half with half-inch meshes. Stones and very hard large lumps would be discharged at the end of the screen; the coarser particles passing through the half-inch mesh might be broken up in a stamping-mill and resifted. If the screening-house were built in a side hill, so that carts could lead directly to the screen, and the prepared earth fall to a story below, much necessity for shovelling would be obviated.

4. Concerning the mechanical arrangement for the Closet, I am more and more inclined to the opinion that Mr. Moule's device is the only one that will be effective under all circumstances. Possibly variations in the size of the "chucker" (by which the quantity of earth used is measured), according to the quality of the earth, may be found to be

desirable. Whether this apparatus is used or whether we depend on covering with a hand-scoop, the quantity should be regulated by the quantity of urine to be absorbed, and at each urination earth should be thrown down, to prevent undue moisture.

In an ordinary broad vault the deposits will naturally form a heap under the seat. This must be, now and then, levelled off, and the surface exposed by the levelling should be thinly covered with the drier earth near the sides of the vault. Probably under no ordinary circumstances would it be necessary to do this oftener than twice in a month. In the commode and the up-stairs closet it will never be necessary. With the Broadmoor tank, or larger vault, it will be.

5. Just as it is requisite to empty a cess-pool, or fill the tank over a water-closet, as occasion requires, so it is necessary to supply fresh earth to the Earth-Closet, and carry away the accumulation. I have shown (page 36) how this is done in the case of a Commode in constant use. Larger closets require a larger amount of labor at one time, but at much longer intervals. The details of this work are too simple to need attention here.

In the case of towns, where the system is in anything like general use, the care of the closets should devolve almost exclusively upon associations or individuals engaged in the business of earth supply. Having, as a gardener, undertaken this in Newport for the sake of the manure to be obtained, I am already convinced that in all places where manure has even a moderate value, it will be unnecessary to make a charge for the earth and attendance. The preparation of the earth and the amount of transportation constitute a trifling tax when compared with the value of the product. When the business increases, so that the time of a man and a horse and cart will be constantly employed, the details can be somewhat simplified, and the rounds made with more regularity; the only precaution necessary being, to have always an abundant supply of earth ready in advance, so that protracted wet weather will not require regular delivery to be postponed in order to make use of the first fair weather for securing earth.

The Dry Earth Company of New Haven have adopted the rule of

charging a moderate price for the first supply of earth, exchanging it without cost whenever necessary. This is done to prevent the use of the manure by householders. Wherever the demand is sufficient for the business to be regularly systematized, the earth may be delivered as ordered, just as coal is now delivered from coal-yards, and it would be proper to make a charge for "carrying in," as in handling coal. If the cart is suitably covered against rain, it is most convenient to carry the earth in bags. These may be emptied into a bin in the cellar, from which commode-hods are supplied, or into the hoist-box of the up-stairs closets, or they may be carried to closets on the upper floors of houses.

The deposits may be removed in baskets, and emptied into the cart on its returning rounds. Barrels are too heavy for one man to handle, and are less convenient than bags for filling closet-reservoirs.

In places where manure has not sufficient value to pay the cost of attendance, the charge necessary to make a profitable business of attending to a considerable number of closets would be much less than the water rates and plumbers' bills that are an inseparable part of the water system. If ashes are used, the addition of the closet manure to them will not materially increase the cost of their handling, and it will give them a value which they do not now possess.

6. In the country where the manure is to be applied directly to the garden, it will be better to use the earth but once, as there is an advantage in having it as bulky as possible for more even distribution; but even in this case it should not be applied in its fresh state. It should be first thrown into a bin or into barrels, in which it will retain its moisture long enough for perfect fermentation. In this way its paper will be destroyed, and its fæcal matter will be diffused throughout the mass and absorbed by the earth; while the earth itself will have its own fertilizing constituents developed by the decomposition going on within it. When ready for use, the earth will be nearly indistinguishable from that freshly taken from the field; but its manurial power will be very much increased. If the manure is to be sold in the market or is to be transported to any distance, it should be repeatedly used, in

order that its value may be as much as possible increased. The deposits taken from the closets should be carried to the earth depot, thrown into compact heaps, moistened a little, if necessary, and left to ferment. After a sufficient time, these heaps may be shovelled over, and left to undergo a second fermentation. They may then be spread out to dry, or, better, removed to a drying-room where there is a free circulation of air. After becoming dry, the earth may be passed through a screen, and the finer parts stored away for further use; the small amount of coarser matter may be again moistened and fermented. Of this latter, the quantity will be very small, and it will consist chiefly of dried-up solid fæces, which it may be found best to pulverize and use directly as manure, or it may be mixed with deposits freshly brought in from the closets. It will help the fermentation of these, and will be entirely absorbed.

There are no data from which the value added to the earth by its use can be definitely fixed. It would vary considerably, according to the kind of earth used and the richness of the food of the people.

7. What is the best arrangement for towns and villages it is now too early to say; but in any case the details of the system would be simple and easy of execution. If the value of the manure is enough to make the earth business a source of profit, it may be safely left to private enterprise; but even in this case the sanitary authorities of the town should provide for the inspection of closets, especially among the poorer classes, and it should be required that all comply with such provisions as the public interest makes necessary.

If the preservation of the manure is not an object, the removal of the accumulations may be provided for, as is now done in the case of ashes, etc. The public authorities should, in all cases, assume such control of the matter as to ensure the perfect working of the system; but the manner in which private establishments shall be supplied with earth is a question to be decided by the peculiar circumstances of each case. Just as no water-closet should be allowed to remain in use without a supply of water or with an obstructed soil-pipe, so should no Earth-Closet be allowed to become ineffective from the neglect of its owner to provide it with earth or to have its accumulations removed. It is now necessary, in even the smallest towns, to prevent any outrageous neglect of common privies; and the extension of the same system of inspection to meet the requirements of the dry-earth sewage would be neither difficult for the authorities nor onerous to householders.

Of course, in large and compactly built cities the amount of governmental control and supervision would have to be greater in proportion to the extent of the population. Many depots for the supply and remanipulation of the earth would be necessary, and everything in connection with the working of the system would demand the most careful attention of officers charged with the preservation of public health. As, however, the duties involved would be very much less than in the case of water supply and foul-water sewage, they need constitute no objection to the adoption of the Earth System.

It would be worth while to experiment on a somewhat extensive scale with a mixture of the ordinary street dirt, coal-ashes, and garbage of the city. It is not unlikely that, if these materials were thrown together and allowed to undergo a single fermentation, they would become, in being dried and sifted, a satisfactory medium of disinfection in closets. If this plan were successful, the cost of importing earth would be entirely obviated, and the enormous refuse, whose removal is now a serious tax, would have given to it a value that would more than counterbalance all cost of manipulation and removal.

THE PHILOSOPHY OF THE EARTH SYSTEM.

HAVING made an earnest effort to discover the precise manner in which the earth that is used to cover and absorb offensive organic matters exercises its influence upon them, I regret to say that it has been impossible to arrive at any satisfactory conclusion with reference to it. An enquiry addressed to Professor S. W. Johnson, of Yale College, brought the following reply:

"The chemistry of the Earth-Closet is not sufficiently understood. "We know something of it. There is oxidation and, under proper con- "ditions, nitrification; but new studies are absolutely required before the "subject can be intelligently discussed. What we now know is just "enough to make further research inviting and easy."

In the "Journal of the Chemical Society of London," series 2, vol. vi., there is an article by Robert Warrington, Jr., on "The part taken "by oxide of iron and alumina in the absorptive action of soils," which describes a series of experiments that seem to prove conclusively that the metallic oxides in the soil help to fix the compound results of putrefaction by actually decomposing them.

Professor J. T. Way, when chemist to the Royal Agricultural Society of England, made investigations on the power of soils to absorb manure, which clearly established a very strong action, either chemical or physical, between the alumina of the soil and various products of organic decomposition.

Professor Way attributes the effect to the double silicates of alumina and some other base, that are found in all clays, and describes a decomposition of these double silicates by the alkaline products of the decomposition of organic matter. He thus explains the action that takes place:

"I have avoided giving any detailed technical account of these

" salts, and have only mentioned those particulars in their history which " bear upon the agricultural question. It is necessary, however, to " notice some points in relation to them as a class. In the first place, " it will have been observed that there is a regular order of decomposi- " tion between the silicates of each base and ordinary salts of other " bases; thus, the soda silicate is decomposed by salts of either lime, " potash, or ammonia; the potash silicate, again, is decomposed in its " turn by lime or ammonia; and, lastly, the lime compound by am- " monia. The different bases may be arranged in the order in which " they replace each other from the silicate, as follows:

" Soda,
" Potash,
" Lime,
" Magnesia,
" Ammonia.

" That is to say, that from a silicate of alumina and any one of " these bases the base will be dislodged by a salt of any of those " under it in the list. Nitrate of potash, for instance, will turn out " soda from its silicate, and a potash silicate will be formed; whilst " ammonia will replace any of the other bases. Of course, the re- " verse of this action cannot occur, and therefore the double silicate of " alumina and ammonia cannot be decomposed by any neutral salt of " the other alkalies."

The following extracts are taken from Dr. Robert Angus Smith's work on " Disinfectants and Disinfection:"

" Animal matter, which chiefly is found to be dangerous, is, in fact, " the fæces or *dejecta* of human beings and of cattle. It might be sup- " posed that these substances had already been decomposed, but such is " not the case. The decomposition is very imperfect, and when they are " allowed to stand putrefaction sets in, closely allied to, perhaps exactly " the same, as that which takes place in other animal matters, such as " blood, or in a mixture of flesh and water. When these substances de- " compose, the result is, so far as we know, nearly the same as the decom- " position of the entire animal body. We are not able to tell the differ- " ence between the products of putrefaction from our cess-pools and " those from our graveyards. The problem, then, of preserving meat, or " of preserving the entire animal from corruption, and the problem of " preserving sewage and fæces from decomposition, become entirely one " and the same. We are required to do for the fæces that which the

" Egyptians did for their bodies, until they shall be thrown upon the " ground, and mixed with the soil and become the food of plants. . . .

" Every substance in fine powder disinfects—dust of all kinds, " whether platinum powder or powder of sandstone. The surface is " enormously increased in such bodies, and surfaces attract the air, which " is confined and pressed into service, causing more active oxidation, and " therefore more purification. . . .

" Pettenkofer says that carbolic acid preserves inert the ferment " cells, but when it is removed they become active. If this is true, the " disinfectant must be used continuously, and the impure matter must be " cleared away continuously, whilst soon in time, *and especially in the " earth*, the infectious matter will die. . . .

" One may very correctly look on the soil as the greatest agent for " purifying and disinfecting. Every impurity is thrown on it in abund- " ance, and yet it is pure, and the breathing of air having the odor of " the soil has, on what exact evidence I do not know, but very generally, " been considered wholesome. . . .

" We desire to prevent from decomposition the manure, from which " it is the problem of Europe to escape. It produces a class of disease " which we generate and foster at home, and assists its relations when " they come, like cholera, to visit it from abroad. . . .

" At present there are two plans: one is to overwhelm with water, " and to carry off in unseen underground streams; another, is to leave " the material as dry as possible, the moisture having been drained and " passed into the atmosphere or the soil. The first mentioned, the " water-closet system, is a great luxury unquestionably, but, like luxuries, " it is taxed. Water is the most powerful agent of infection known to us " as well as of disinfection. Substances which preserve for ever dry, be- " come putrid at once when moist. All organic bodies decompose most " rapidly in it, and if it is sent out of our towns laden with riches, it " rapidly dissipates them all and sends them into the air. It is the " very symbol of abundance and extravagance. Manure will not keep " in it, and will not carry in it long. Cess-pools, which were deposits of " manure and water, were found after much loss of life to be manufac- " turers of disease of the most active nature, and water-closets which are " not carefully attended to obtain an odor by no means agreeable. . . .

" The action of water in removing deleterious substances is partly " mechanical; it lifts or makes lighter particles not easily reached, and " the impure matter is diffused through the liquid to be oxidized without " necessarily evaporating. Without it, it seems impossible to produce "absolute purity of surface in most cases. When it is saturated, however, it begins to give off vapors into the atmosphere, and, as water may be said to be equal to a porous body having an unlimited surface, its activity is very great. It absorbs oxygen rapidly, helps it to oxidize the organic matter, and send forth carbonic acid, and along with it many vapors into the atmosphere, and intensifies the operation to such an extent that bodies which would have lain in a mass for years undecomposed are, where mixed with water in a moving stream, completely rendered invisible in a few days. This has been found in a remarkable case in which the sewage of a large town, moving slowly after being mixed with an immense excess of water, has been found utterly to disappear, so that only the slightest trace of soluble matter of an organic origin could be found in it. Even the deposit, gradually diminishing, had ceased to be offensive, the ammonia, which was nearly a grain per gallon to begin with, could not at last be discovered; whilst the evaporation seems to have gone on in warmish weather at the rate of one grain per square foot daily. Although, therefore, water is a wonderful agent of purification, it is also an agent for the contrary, because it causes a very rapid and effervescing decomposition of organic matter, and, if in enormous quantities, it sends out impure as well as pure gases into the atmosphere. It is for that reason, apparently, that wet cess-pools have been found so dangerous, and that stagnant pools are also dreaded."

Professor Charles A. Joy, of Columbia College, in an article on "Earth-Closets," * says:

"The diisnfecting property of dry earth, humus, clay, charcoal, peat, bone-black, ashes, and other solid substances, has long been known, and all of these bodies have been applied in one way and another for the prevention of bad odors, for the filtration of water and absorption of gases. The bodies of the dead have, with most nations, been buried beneath the soil, and thus all danger likely to arise during their decay has been removed.

"In the thickly populated regions of the East, necessity has impelled the inhabitants to have recourse to the same principle in the disinfecting of all fæcal matter; but in a sparsely settled country great carelessness is apt to creep in and to maintain its supremacy, long after a large increase of population imperatively demands as much

* *The Journal of Applied Chemistry*, January, 1870.

" care in the removal of all excremental matter as it does in the proper " disposition of dead bodies.

" The action of dry earth is not only chemical but physical, and " consists mainly in the absorption and removal of the water necessary to " the decay of organic substances; the formation of dangerous gases is " thus prevented, and the animal matter is left to a slow decay (combus- " tion) and no odors can arise.

" A small amount of earth is sufficient to disinfect a considerable " quantity of putrid or offensive matter, and for this reason its use has " been strongly recommended in hospitals in cases of bad sores and " wounds.

" The recent learned researches of Pettenkofer on the causes of " typhus and cholera have led to the conclusion that these dangerous " diseases prevail in regions where the water from sewers, out-houses, " sinks, etc., approaches near the surface. In fact, the cholera was " traced along the water-courses, and the upper part of the same valley " would be left untouched, while the lower portions were subjected to " the ravages of the disease. During a dry season the disease was less " likely to appear than during a wet. The incontrovertible conclusion " forced itself upon the mind of Pettenkofer that there was nothing more " dangerous than to have the water near a dwelling contaminated by " the diseased fæcal excreta of the population, and he sought for some " remedy for this startling evil. If he had heard of the epidemic in the " National Hotel at Washington, and of the fever that proved so fatal " at the Pittsfield Seminary, he would have had some further confirma- " tion of the accuracy of this theory.

" The labors of Pettenkofer in Germany have been ably seconded " by those of the Rev. Henry Moule, of Fordington Vicarage, Dorset- " shire, England. He experimented with a large number of sub- " stances, and finally returned to mother earth, where he found, in the " cheapest of all material, the very best agent for the removal of " danger.

" He proposed to use dry earth as a disinfectant, and invented a " simple contrivance for the application of this principle to Commodes, " thus doing away with all out-houses and other sources of evil about " the homestead.

" If his suggestions could be universally applied, there is no doubt " that the death-rate from typhus, intermittent fever, and cholera " would be greatly reduced, and the general health of every family " largely promoted. . . .

" The advantages and importance of Earth-Closets must be ap-
" parent to every one who has followed us thus far in our article. They " require very little architectural change, and can be put anywhere " when a vault is not already dug; they are entirely without odor, and " preserve in the best way the full agricultural value of the manure.

" If there is a suitable room about the premises for the construction " of the reservoir for the earth, it can be made sufficiently large to re- " quire to be rarely filled. Where there is a scarcity of earth, it is better " to dry and use it several times. The contents of the hod must, in this " event, be carried daily to a particular spot, and there dried and sifted. " In warm climates this can easily be done, but in wet seasons some " artificial method for drying must be employed. Twenty-four cubic " inches of earth are probably enough for each drop, or a cubic foot for " seventy-two times; at the rate of 400 visits per annum for each per- " son, the yearly consumption would be five and a half cubic feet of " earth; and where the earth is used eight times over, the requirements " would be about one cubic foot per annum for each person. This " estimate shows that the labor of providing all of the necessary earth " must be very small in the country, and it is probable that, after a few " years, the rich compost will become a source of profit, and the earth " will cost nothing.

" Surely, a system that will save many lives, keep up the good " health of the family, avoid waste of valuable manure, and is cheap and " easy of application, ought to be universally substituted for the waste- " ful, dangerous, unhealthy custom handed down to us by our fore- " fathers."

TESTIMONY

IN FAVOR OF THE

EARTH-CLOSET.

THE NOVELTY IRON WORKS in New York City occupy eight acres of ground, and employ about one thousand men. Their water-tax on water-closets was $1,500 per annum. To escape this, they propose to take out their forty-eight water-closets and substitute the same number of Earth-Closets. After six months' trial, with nine fixed Closets, they give the following opinion of their value:

Office of THE NOVELTY IRON WORKS,
NEW YORK, Dec. 28, 1869.

We have now given the Earth-Closet a thorough trial, and can say that it gives *entire satisfaction*. I do not hesitate to recommend it for manufactories, machine-shops, etc., as in every respect superior to the water-closet.

W. P. TROWBRIDGE, VICE-PRESIDENT.

UNIVERSITY OF PENNSYLVANIA, MEDICAL DEPARTMENT,
PHILADELPHIA, Jan. 5, 1870.

I have used the Earth-Closet obtained from you in my private room in the University, since last October, with entire satisfaction.

I regard it not only as a great convenience, but as an equally great hygienic improvement, and, where water-closets cannot be constructed, as a valuable and complete substitute for them.

FRANCIS G. SMITH, M.D.

LAKE FOREST, ILL.,
Dec. 24, 1869.

We, the undersigned, having used your Commodes for several months, and having given them as severe a test as they need ever be subjected to, take pleasure in testifying to their satisfactory working, and to the perfect deodorizing properties of fine Dry Earth. For use either in public buildings or private residences we consider them preferable to water-closets, as being *entirely free from odor.*

E. P. WESTON, PRINCIPAL LAKE FOREST FEMALE SEMINARY.
IRA W. ALLEN, PRINCIPAL LAKE FOREST ACADEMY.
E. S. SKINNER, SECRETARY LAKE FOREST UNIVERSITY.
WILLIAM WARREN, WESTERN MANAGER LONDON, LIVERPOOL, AND GLOBE INSURANCE CO.

FORT ADAMS, NEWPORT, R. I.
Dec. 15, 1869.

A number of Commodes and fixtures for Earth-Closets have been in use by the garrison of Fort Adams for several months past, and have given entire satisfaction, *completely answering the purpose for which they are designed.* The application of the Earth-Closet principle is of the highest importance as regards convenience, health, and economy. It does away with a great nuisance, and enables us to utilize a most valuable fertilizer at a trifling outlay. The Commodes can be placed wherever needed for convenience—a great advantage in cases of sickness and in hospitals. It is only necessary to follow the few simple directions for their use to appreciate their advantages. *The Soldiers' Closet works perfectly.*

D. C. HOUSTON,
MAJOR U. S. ENGINEERS, BREVET COL. U. S. A.

BALTIMORE, MD., October 9, 1869.

The Earth-Closet in my establishment is a complete success, and it supplies a great want which, in this and thousands of other cases, it is difficult to meet in any other way.

W. F. DAILY, SURGICAL INSTRUMENT FACTORY,
243 West Baltimore Street.

WEST HAVEN, CONN., NOV. 19, 1869.

A few months ago I purchased one of Rev. Henry Moule's Patent Commodes or Earth-Closets, and although I had some doubts at the time in regard to its deodorizing and disinfecting qualities being as represented, yet I find, by a most careful test, that it has more than justified your recommendation. I have had sickness in my family, and the Commode has been thoroughly tested, and I would not now part with it for the price of three if I was unable to get another. Respectfully yours, etc.,

CHANDLER FOSTER.

We take great pleasure in testifying our entire satisfaction with the practical operation of the Earth-Closet erected at our new works, The Closet is located in the lower part of the main building, in close contiguity to a passage-way daily used by many persons, and is so entirely odorless that we are quite sure few, if any, have ever suspected its design.

SAVAGE & KEYSER, CHEMICAL WORKS,
Philadelphia, Pa.

MEDICAL DIRECTOR'S OFFICE,
DEPARTMENT OF THE EAST,
NEW YORK CITY, Dec. 15, 1869.

I have carefully examined and studied the system of Earth-Closets, and have, on all proper occasions urgently recommended the system to be adopted in our army hospitals and barracks. I am well satisfied that this system, when thoroughly understood, will be generally resorted to, even where water is at command.

JOHN M. CUYLER,
SURGEON & BREVET BRIG. GEN. U. S. A.

BOSTON, Dec. 20, 1869.

Everything which concerns the health, comfort, and welfare of the people is a matter of interest to me, as it should be to every other person. I therefore commend the Earth-Closet system as, in my judgment, the most important sanitary discovery of the age, simple in its arrangement, sure in its operation, and beneficent in its results. A careful examination of it is very certain to induce a trial of it, and the trial is equally certain to sustain all that is claimed for it. Its merits need only to be known to procure for it the widest demand. Indeed, I think no commendation of it can be too strongly expressed. "Eureka" should be its motto or trade-mark. There should be at least one Earth-Commode in every household, for its signal convenience and utility, especially in cases of sickness, it being as easily removed from room to room as a chair or a table, and very neatly constructed as a piece of furniture. The one I purchased fulfils all my expectations.

WILLIAM LLOYD GARRISON.

NEW YORK, December 22, 1869.

If I had known before leaving England that these closets were procurable here, I should not have brought over the four I imported, as my sole object was to propagate here, by their introduction, knowledge of an invention which so perfectly accomplishes its purpose that I felt sure, if once known, it must take.

It may interest you to know that my attention was first attracted to the Earth-Closet system by finding at an English country-seat, where I was visiting, Earth-Closets in use up-stairs and down, although the house, a handsome and well-appointed one, had water-closets on the same floors. The fact was so striking, and my host spoke so highly of the Earth-Closets, that I informed myself further about them, and decided to bring some out to this country.

I hope you will meet with all success; for, whether regard is had to economy, health, or decency, the Earth-Closet is, *facile princeps*, beating the water-closet decidedly on the first two points, and the every way offensive system which is in common use here in the country on all three.

I am yours faithfully,

HOWARD POTTER.

GLENBROOK FARM, WEST HAVERFORD, PA,
October 20, 1869.

It gives me pleasure to endorse, from my own experience, both the *principle and the practical operations of your Earth-Closets.* The fixtures I purchased from you in August last I have had put up under an enclosed porch immediately at my office door, and *within ten feet of my desk.* So far from finding it in any way offensive or unpleasant, I consider it *one of the greatest improvements I have added to my house.* Wishing you success in your efforts to introduce the system generally,

I remain yours truly,

JOHN R. WHITNEY.

Letter from Dr. R. S. Stewart, President of the Maryland Hospital, Baltimore.

MARYLAND HOSPITAL, Aug. 1, 1869.

I believe I have given the Earth-Closet a full and fair trial, and can now say without hesitation that I think it is an invention of the greatest importance to society generally.

It does all that you claim for it; and I have no doubt it will in a great degree supersede water-closets and common privies.

Its cheapness is one of its greatest advantages, for it can be obtained by families of the humblest means, securing to them a degree of domestic comfort and health unknown heretofore to all excepting the rich who can afford to have water-closets in their establishments.

It is less liable to injury and to get out of order, and more easily repaired when it does. Besides, it saves without trouble or expense the most valuable manure for the farm and garden.

I therefore recommend it to my fellow-citizens as one of the most important inventions of the age.

R. S. STEWART, PREST. MARYLAND HOSPITAL.

ST. MARK'S SCHOOL, SOUTHBOROUGH, MASS., Jan. 13, 1870.

I will give you my unhesitating and unreserved testimony to the absolute excellence of the Dry Earth System.

ROBERT LOWELL.

The following was written for the *American Agricultural Annual*, 1870, by Col. M. C. Weld.

The very important bearing this subject has upon agriculture led the writer to look carefully into it several years since, and more than three years ago the Earth-Closet was an "institution" in his family economy, introduced notwithstanding many doubts, and retained as an indispensable comfort. We heartily wish all dwellers in the country, who daily and nightly are obliged to subject themselves, and the ladies of their families, to the exposure of a walk of several rods to reach a retreat, secluded under vines and behind hollyhocks, perhaps, but oftener open to the broad glare of day and the eyes of the passer or the curious, could have the same comfort. However secluded, the conventional privy is an abomination which, after a few years, we shall wonder was ever endured in the latter half of the nineteenth century.

The Earth-Closet, supplied constantly with dry earth, is odorless and neat. It may be in the house or in the wood-shed. It is well to have it where it may be entered unobserved, and so arranged that dry earth may be brought in and removed without attracting attention.

ALBANY, N. Y., Jan. 20, 1870.

In reply to your request for my opinion of the Dry Earth Commode, I am able to speak most unequivocally in its favor.

One has been in constant use in my house for several months, and is regarded as an indispensable convenience. Doubtless, arguments in favor of the water-closet system will be offered against the Dry Earth System, *but simplicity, economy, and science must determine a verdict in favor of the latter.*

In the marvellous process of disintegration and renewal throughout the animal and vegetable worlds, a constant demand is created in one organization for those products which are eliminated from another organization as effete or useless. In the Dry Earth System, this fact is regarded, and the fertilizing constituents of the flesh and vegetables which we eat, after playing their part in the human economy, are conveniently and inoffensively preserved for the use of the farmer and the gardener in those beautiful laboratories whose chemical products are the flower, the fruit, and the grain. Yours truly,

C. A. ROBERTSON, M.D.

BOSTON COLLEGE, Dec. 21, 1869.

From experiments which I had ordered as President of the College of the Holy Cross, Worcester, Mass., I was convinced that "Earth-Closets" and the "Earth System" were among the most useful discoveries of the age. Your obedient servant,

R. W. BRADY, S.J.

UNION COLLEGE, SCHENECTADY, N. Y.,
Dec. 29, 1869.

. . . I am, as I expected to be, perfectly satisfied as to their value and efficacy. Respectfully,

(Professor) MAURICE PERKINS.

Extract from the Report of the Massachusetts State Board of Health.

EARTH CLOSETS.

"This is one of the simplest and yet one of the most useful discoveries of modern times.

"Hereafter, if we are wise, we shall apply this simple means for the purification of vaults in every place where water is not used for that purpose, as in our great cities.

"In the country it will be invaluable; and whenever in private houses cholera or typhoid fever, or any contagious disease, may occur, there should this principle involved in the Earth-Closet be adopted."

WESTBORO, MASS., Jan. 4, 1870.

We have been using your Earth-Closets for the last three weeks, and have been much pleased with them.

The principle upon which they act is simple, yet effective. The amount of dry earth or ashes scattered over the deposits seems to deodorize it so that nothing offensive escapes. Should they continue to give satisfaction (and I see no reason why they should not), I shall recommend a more extended use of them to the Board of Trustees. Your Commodes must be very convenient for family use and invaluable for the sick-room. Yours very truly,

BENJAMIN EVANS,
SUPERINTENDENT STATE REFORM SCHOOL.

NEWPORT, R. I., Jan. 7, 1870.

Most willingly do I comply with your request to give you the result of my experience with the Earth-Closet. I am glad to contribute my mite towards making known its efficacy.

The expositions and testimonials contained in your circulars so satisfied me of the reality of the discovery that *dry clay* is a deodorizer of fæces, that some months ago, as you are aware, I set up in the basement of my house a closet with a self-acting apparatus, furnished by your Company.

It were not enough to say that the experiment has been successful; the success has surpassed expectation. It proves that in dry, sifted clay there is a virtue by means of which the refuse of the human body is so taken hold of that it is reconverted into inoffensive earth. The reservoir is emptied into barrels which stand just outside of the door of the closet, and, although uncovered, there is from them no smell whatever. In these barrels there is not only the best fertilizer for the garden or farm, but one which can be handled with as much cleanliness as though the barrels were filled with sod and earth. It seems to me that this discovery may be turned into a manifold and wide benefaction through its perfect healthfulness, its cleanliness, and the saving of so much fertilizing material. Truly yours,

G. H. CALVERT.

CONNECTICUT STATE HOSPITAL,
NEW HAVEN, Dec. 22, 1869.

The Earth-Closets and Commodes furnished by you have been in use in this hospital for the past six months. They continue to work satisfactorily, and are daily demonstrating their usefulness. *The deposit is completely deodorized, and is no more offensive to the sight or smell than an equal quantity of coal-ashes.*

Very truly yours,

L. D. WILCOXSON, M.D.

NEW HAVEN, CONN., Jan. 3, 1870.

We concur in the opinion of Dr. Wilcoxson, and beg leave to add that no greater convenience has been added to the hospital during our connection with the institution.

W. G. ALLING, RESIDENT PHYSICIAN.
JOSEPH COLTON, STEWARD.

RAHWAY, NEW JERSEY, April 15, 1869.

I take the pleasure of saying that the Moule's Patent Commode . . . has proved in every way satisfactory; in fact, since we have had it in use, we would not be without it. *We consider it in many respects superior to the stationary water-closet in the house.*

In a sick-room it is indispensable, and, once introduced in any household, I think it will, as it eminently deserves, become a permanent piece of furniture. Respectfully yours,

JOHN F. WHITING, MAYOR.

SCHENECTADY, N. Y., Dec. 20, 1869.

I have had the form of the Earth-Closet known as the Commode in constant use for the past two months. It being difficult to procure dry earth so late in the season, I have substituted for it sifted anthracite coal-ashes.

The Commode has worked well in all respects, and the ashes seem to be as perfect a deodorizer and disintegrater as can be desired. There is no offensive smell, and the contents of the hod when it is emptied appear to consist of ashes only. I can conceive of no objection that can be urged against the ashes, except that, from its lightness and consequent bulkiness, the hod is sooner filled than if earth were used, and must be emptied more frequently.

If the product is to be used, as it always should be, as a fertilizer, I think the ashes preferable to earth, where the soil to which it is to be applied is heavy. *As to the value of this joint result of discovery and invention, considered in all its relations, sanitary and economical, as promotive of decency and comfort, and supplying an important desideratum for every human habitation, it is impossible to overestimate it.*

Yours truly,

(Professor) J. W. JACKSON.

BOSTON, CITY HALL, Dec. 27, 1869.

As Chairman of the Committee from the Board of Aldermen of this city, appointed to assist at the Jubilee Festival, I had occasion to observe the working of the Earth-Closets, which were placed in the different rooms of the Coliseum in June last by the agent of the Earth-Closet Company, and can say that I heard no criticism of them except that which was favorable, and they appeared to be an entire success.

Truly yours,

EDWARD A. WHITE.

WETHERSFIELD, CONN., April 8, 1869.

The Commode which I received from you three weeks since has been in use in my family from that time, to my perfect satisfaction. Having no dry earth, we have used it with our anthracite coal-ashes, and, although it is in a closet opening directly into one of my family rooms, no one would suspect its being in the house. Yours truly,

S. W. ROBBINS.

BOARD OF HEALTH, OFFICE OF SANITARY SUPERINTENDENT,
CHICAGO, November 30, 1869.

I have for the past three years examined and witnessed the practical working of the Earth-Closet, and am satisfied that under a great variety of circumstances it affords the best means of disposing of night-soil, with reference to both sanitary and economical considerations.

It is particularly valuable in this city, and in all localities where similar conditions obtain with regard to drainage.

JOHN H. RAUCH, Sanitary Superintendent.

Philadelphia, April 10, 1869.

Having tested one of Moule's Patent Earth-Closets (manufactured by the Earth-Closet Company, of Hartford), with my patients in the *Pennsylvania Hospital* in a manner which may fairly be said to have been a very severe one, I am confident that it not only warrants all that is claimed for it, but *fulfils all the requirements of such a convenience for a hospital as well as for a sick-chamber, or for family use.*

ADDINELL HEWSON, M.D.

Professor Samuel W. Johnson, of Yale College, widely known as the leading Agricultural Chemist of the country, writes as follows:

Sheffield Scientific School of Yale College,
New Haven, Conn., March 29, 1869.

I have read your little publication on Earth-Closets with great interest, and am glad to learn that you are taking active measures to bring the subject practically to the notice of our people. I am myself familiar with the use of dry earth as a disinfectant and a drier of fæces. *Nothing can be more instant and effectual than its operation, and its use has every sanitary advantage.*

The agricultural aspect of the subject is of the highest interest and importance. The Earth-Closet enables us to effect a more than Chinese economy of our night-soil and urine, in combination with the utmost cleanliness, convenience, and cheapness.

The Commode of Mr. Moule, as improved by you and manufactured at Hartford, *is very effective and convenient* for hospital and sick-room use, and I trust the public will not be slow to avail themselves of the "Reform" which your enterprise now puts within their reach.

Yours most truly,

S. W. JOHNSON.

Fort Adams, R. I., Jan. 24, 1870.

The system of Earth-Closets at Fort Adams appears to have at length settled a question which for twenty years or more has been a source of infinite perplexity, trouble, and expense.

Early in August last a set of these closets was erected in one of the casemates; and since that time—or nearly six months—they have been in daily use by more than a hundred men. I have closely watched the experiment. *The result is perfectly satisfactory. No odor from the deposit can be detected in the casemate.*

The labor of procuring, drying, and sifting the requisite earth is but trifling, and (apart from the agricultural value of the product) is repaid a thousand-fold by the comfort, safety, and certainty secured in the removal of the excreta, and by relief from the former nuisance of cess-pools and water-closets, which hereafter should never be permitted in a permanent fortification. Very truly yours,

J. F. HEAD, Surgeon U. S. Army.

The following is from the Landscape Architects and Superintendents of the Central Park, New York; Prospect Park, Brooklyn; and Riverside Improvement Company, Illinois :

Office of the Brooklyn Park Commission,
November 20, 1869.

From ten to twenty Earth-Closets have been in constant public use upon the Brooklyn Parks during the last year, under our supervision. *They have more than met our expectations, proving in all respects satisfactory.*

We are now introducing them in *preference* to water-closets, *even where water supply is already secured, and sewers laid.*

Yours, etc.,

OLMSTED VAUX & CO.,
Landscape Architects and Superintendents.

Pacific Mills, Lawrence, Mass., Feb. 11, 1870.

Dear Sir: The eight Earth-Closets which you furnished us for one of our tenements for operatives are working satisfactorily, and I consider them a great addition to the comfort and sanitary condition of a family.

W. C. CHAPIN, Agent Pacific Mills.

www.ingramcontent.com/pod-product-compliance
Lightning Source LLC
LaVergne TN
LVHW021428110826
845150LV00007B/2139

* 9 7 8 1 4 2 5 5 0 6 8 5 8 *